A History of the
WARRNAMBOOL & DISTRICT
BASE HOSPITAL

By GORDON FORTH & PETER YULE

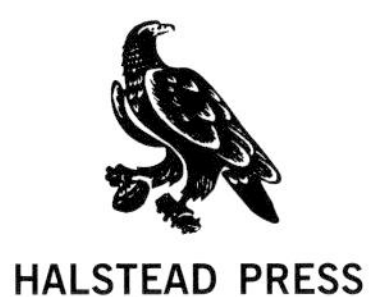

HALSTEAD PRESS

SYDNEY MMII
Published by Halstead Press
19a Boundary Street,
Rushcutters Bay, New South Wales, 2011

 Typeset by Brevier Design, Kensington, N.S.W. Printed by Brown Prior Anderson, Melbourne.

Cataloguing in publication entry data available from the National Library. Call no. 362.11099457

ISBN 1 875684 90 5

Contents

Acknowledgements

The following history of the Warrnambool and District Base Hospital was undertaken by Deakin University's Centre for Regional Development with funding provided by the Hospital's Board of Management. Throughout this project we received every assistance from staff of the Hospital. We should especially like to thank Barbara Piesse, current president of the Hospital Board, Andrew Rowe, the Chief Executive Officer, Sue Morrison, Director of Nursing, Cathy Dalton, Hospital Librarian, and Gary Druitt, Chief Information Officer for South West Association of Rural Hospitals for their much valued contribution to the history. We also wish to express our appreciation for the contributions of former Board President, Mr Frank Lodge, Dr David Shimmin, and Les O'Callaghan, President of Warrnambool Historical Society, for reading the manuscript and offering constructive advice. We should also like to acknowledge the excellent work of Centre project officers Tim Bligh and Penny Forth who conducted interviews and undertook research for the history, and Michelle Jansen, Faculty of Arts, Deakin University, who typed and assisted in the revision of the manuscript. Finally and most importantly we wish to express our gratitude to the individuals who agreed to participate in interviews regarding their first hand experience of the Hospital.

Gordon Forth and Peter Yule

Introduction

The Warrnambool Base Hospital, now South West Healthcare, Warrnambool campus, provides the city's most prominent landmark, which can be observed from many vantage points within Warrnambool. This is highly appropriate, as for most of its history, the "Base" has had a central role in the lives of the residents of both the city and the surrounding region. Generations of local people have been born, given birth, been treated for a range of medical conditions, and died within the Base Hospital precinct. In more recent times the Hospital has extended its ever-increasing range of services into the homes of residents.

The relationship between this hospital and its community has been, and remains, a mutually supportive and intimate one. Given the extent to which Victoria's public hospitals now rely on State Government funding, the degree to which a regional base hospital like Warrnambool's depends on its community for financial and in-kind support should not be underestimated. Since its humble beginnings, the Hospital has always relied on and received outstanding support from its local community. This support has varied, reflecting the Hospital's specific needs at the time and the capabilities of individuals and organisations to contribute to the work of the Hospital. While Warrnambool's prominent citizens gave freely of their time to serve on committees or boards, other groups, such as ladies' auxiliaries and local schools, raised funds for the Hospital through "egg drives", "ugly man competitions" and other equally imaginative initiatives. Clearly this history should provide an account of the Hospital's growth, the construction of new buildings, the purchase of more advanced equipment and the appointment of key staff. It is equally important that the extent of community support that in its various forms made much of this growth possible should also be properly documented.

Throughout most of its long history the Warrnambool and district community understood the critical importance of having a quality public hospital. This understanding is obviously largely due to individuals' awareness of the importance of readily accessible, quality health care for themselves and their families. But it also reflects a well-developed sense of civic pride within this community. It is now generally accepted that if Warrnambool is to retain and improve its standing as one of Victoria's key regional growth centres, it needs to have a quality public hospital. Yet the central importance of the Hospital/South West Healthcare to Warrnambool's and south-west Victoria's future growth has not always been well understood. With the relative decline of Australia's agricultural and manufacturing sectors as generators of wealth and employment, health care, like tourism and education, is a critical part of the region's growing service sector. Given Australia's ageing population the demand for an ever-increasing range of health and related services will continue to rise.

The decision of the Hospital Board in 1998 to commission Deakin University to produce a history of the Hospital was particularly timely. Although the actual date of the establishment of the Base Hospital's precedent institution is unclear, the first recorded meeting of the Warrnambool Benevolent Society, which established the Warrnambool Hospital and Benevolent Asylum, was held in June 1851. The publication of the Hospital's history was intended to be part of its sesquicentenary celebrations in 2001. However, unanticipated delays meant that publication did not take place until May 2002. There are sound reasons why most of Australia's major, long established hospitals have published histories to celebrate major milestones. The association between hospitals and the communities they serve is an intimate one. This is particularly the case in regional centres like Warrnambool, where the Hospital is a major source of local employment and where the staff live as well as work in that centre. In contrast, say, to the history of Melbourne's hospitals, the history of a regional hospital is very much a history of a community as well as an institution. In a regional community like south-west Victoria, the development and maintenance of a public hospital system continue to be key factors in the quality of life of residents as well as in the future prosperity of the community. Although Warrnambool has a quality private hospital, St John of God, in many other regional centres there is no alternative health care provider. Throughout its history Warrnambool's civic leaders have been aware that the town's reputation was closely linked to that of "their" hospital.

The Board's decision to produce and publish a history of the Hospital was made at a time when the institution was undergoing major structural change, with the establishment of South West Healthcare. It is clear that the period when Victoria's public hospitals operated as basically autonomous administrative units has come to an end. The former State Coalition Government's intention was to provide incentives to regional base hospitals to amalgamate or enter into voluntary alliances or networks with other public hospitals. In June 1999 what was formerly Warrnambool Base Hospital (the Base) became the Warrnambool campus of South West Healthcare, which included the former Camperdown and Lismore District Hospitals. The Base is now also part of an information technology driven South West Voluntary Alliance of Rural Hospitals, consisting of 14 public hospitals, the largest unit in an information technology linked health care region which includes hospitals as far apart as Apollo Bay and Casterton. These recent initiatives are part of continuing development towards a highly integrated system of regional health care. What was the Warrnambool and District

Base Hospital is now part of several regional hospital networks, which collectively have responsibility for providing quality, cost efficient care for the region. This development parallels south-west Victoria's evolution as a wider political, economic and service region. As a region with considerable human and natural resources, yet in overall decline in demographic terms, the south-west's future growth will in part depend on the willingness of previously autonomous rural centres and institutions, including public hospitals, to act cooperatively. Without this cooperation local health care providers' capacity to provide a broad range of cost efficient services will be limited. Put simply, with a total catchment population of around 100,000, the region has the capacity to provide all but the most specialised health services.

Clearly this evolution has affected the close and mutually supportive relationship that the former base and district hospitals had with the towns and district communities in which they were located. Regardless of the arguments in favour of or against such, changes, the Base has come to the end of its history as a town and district hospital. Thus it is particularly timely to produce a published record of the Hospital's history, from its humble origins as a charitable institution providing basic residential care for Warrnambool's aged poor and destitute, to its development as one of Australia's outstanding regional hospitals.

As there would be with any institution there have been a number of difficulties in producing a balanced, accurate and comprehensive account of the Hospital's development from the early 1850s to the late 1990s. This is partly because of the decision to extend the history to the present. While authors can afford to libel the dead, and need not fear offending them, this is not the case with the living. Extending the Hospital's history to the present day involves legal and ethical considerations. It is quite usual to include in institutional histories details of scandals and serious personality conflicts which occurred several decades ago. However, one has to be much more cautious in describing similar incidents which directly or indirectly involve living persons. This is not only a matter of "good taste" but necessary if authors and publishers wish to avoid litigation. As with most hospital histories, much of the information in this book regarding the past 50 years was obtained through personal interviews—with former patients and staff, current board members and employees and local medical practitioners. As part of Deakin University's required research procedures, formal ethical agreements were negotiated with all individuals who agreed to be interviewed. In the course of certain interviews requests were made that specific comments were to be regarded as "off the record". Interviewees were also provided with an opportunity to check, amend and approve transcripts of their interview. As a further safeguard, the late Dr Kevin Longton, Dr David Shimmin former hospital board president, Frank Lodge and Les O'Callaghan agreed to read and comment on the draft manuscript.

Given these ethical and professional constraints we have sought to produce a truthful, balanced and readable account of the life of this hospital. To make it as relevant as possible to potential readers, including current, former and future patients and staff, we sought to focus on people rather than on buildings and policies. While not wishing to reveal confidences or give offence, we saw no point in producing another bland commemorative institutional history. Such commissioned histories of local government, schools and hospitals understandably remain largely unread. One insults the reader's intelligence to pretend that the Warrnambool Base Hospital, a complex institution like any other, has somehow avoided organisational tension and professional and personal conflicts that are part of institutional life.

While ethical considerations were of some concern in writing recent history, a major difficulty in completing its early history was a general lack of primary sources. This was particularly the case in the Hospital's foundation period. It is unfortunate that the early records of Warrnambool Benevolent Society had been lost or destroyed by the time Richard Osburne wrote his detailed history of Warrnambool in 1887. For much of the Heytesbury/Warrnambool Hospital and Benevolent Asylum's early history, we have only been able to provide a very general account with significant gaps. There were also difficulties in documenting the Hospital's history during the second half of the nineteenth century. Unlike a modern Australian hospital which operates within a highly regulated environment, hospitals in the nineteenth century were the responsibility of a local committee of management. As a consequence, there is little that can be said about the relative quality of the Hospital's care of patients or management of the institution's finances. One area where Warrnambool Hospital appears to have been superior to other country hospitals was the general quality of doctors who worked as honorary medical officers. As a pleasant seaside town located within reasonable proximity to Melbourne, Warrnambool was able to attract and retain the services of such gifted medical practitioners as Drs Jamieson, Fleetwood and Singleton. In time these individuals together with capable administrative and nursing staff enabled Warrnambool to develop a reputation for a good country hospital, a factor which has been significant in enabling the institution to attract and retain quality medical staff and strong support from its community.

Yet while Warrnambool Hospital in the late nineteenth century had several outstanding medical practitioners, caution needs to be exercised in making any general assessment of local doctors' claims regarding qualifications and memberships of professional associations, given that the main source of this information was advertisements placed by doctors themselves in local newspapers.

While available sources relating to the Hospital's more recent past are comprehensive and detailed, they do not always provide a balanced account of the Hospital's development. Put simply, much of the primary source material, including the transcripts of interviews with former patients, staff and local medical practitioners, tends to emphasise the Hospital's undoubted achievements rather than difficulties experienced by the institution. This is most obvious in the Hospital's annual reports which quite properly seek to reassure government and the local community that it's affairs are being well managed. The coverage of major developments in the recent history of the Hospital by the *Standard* are for the most part celebratory rather than critical in tone. Items in the *Standard* are usually based on information provided by the Hospital in the form of press releases or interviews with the CEO or other senior staff. However the *Standard* in its coverage of controversial developments, such as the closure of Brierly Hospital or reductions in Government funding for the Hospital, provided an important forum for public discussion. The *Standard*'s letters to the editor page has provided local residents with the opportunity to publicly criticise as well as endorse the work of the Hospital. Controversial incidents, such as when the local Right to Life movement held night vigils in protest against the use of Hospital facilities to terminate unwanted pregnancies, generated a stream of lively correspondence in the *Standard*.

In writing an account of the Hospital's history since the 1930s, some of the most valuable information came from interviews conducted by Penny Forth with former, usually elderly, patients, current and former staff, board members and local medical practitioners who have or had a professional association with the Hospital. In the case of the former patients who agreed to be interviewed, most were highly appreciative of the care they received. Where former patients were critical of the Hospital, a number requested that such comments be regarded as "off the record". In the case of the local doctors who were interviewed, what was significant was their consistent view of the Base as an outstanding regional hospital. It should be pointed out that (with one exception) we did not interview individuals who could be described as disgruntled former patients or employees of the Hospital. Nor did we consider it appropriate to arrange interviews with patients who had been admitted to the Hospital since 1972.

In the initial negotiations between Deakin University and the Hospital regarding this project it was agreed that our aim would be to produce a balanced, hence interesting, history rather than a commemorative account. We perhaps also needed to take into account the background of the authors, both of whom are long term Warrnambool residents. As professional historians we are obliged to maintain a sense of detachment. However it is not possible to live in a regional community like Warrnambool for over twenty years without absorbing something of this community's strongly developed sense of pride in the city's achievements. As long term residents whose children were born at the Base, it was particularly satisfying to us when the research revealed that Warrnambool Base has been for some decades, one of Australia's outstanding regional hospitals. However in spite of the obstacles which confronted us, we have sought to produce a history that is essentially honest as well as readable.

Chapter 1

FOUNDATION

In 1844 Tom Browne (better known by his pseudonym of Rolf Boldrewood), while travelling west to set up a new cattle station, camped for about six months near the mouth of the Merri River. He described how he went "riding down to the shore one bright day, just below where Warrnambool now stands. No trace of man or habitation was there."[1] Less than three years after Tom Browne enjoyed the solitude of Lady Bay, the first Warrnambool land sales were held. By the end of 1847 a flourishing township was established. The census of 1850 showed the population of Warrnambool as 342, and in that year, within three years of the first settlement of the town, the first moves were made which led to formation of a hospital.

Warrnambool owed its development to the fertility of its hinterland. By the early 1850s the farms to the north and west of Warrnambool grew a large proportion of Victoria's wheat, as well as large quantities of potatoes, onions and other major crops. The staples of more recent years—beef, wool and dairy products—have always been important, but less so in the nineteenth century than today. Farming in the 1850s was highly labour intensive, and in the absence of transport, farm workers had to live close to their employment, so the population of the surrounding districts grew very rapidly. The site of Koroit was still forest in 1856, but in 1870 the township became a borough. Many places which are now just names on the map, such as Ballangeich, or have just a few houses left, like Ellerslie, were substantial villages in the second half of the nineteenth century, with shops, schools, and churches. However, few villages had doctors and only Warrnambool and Port Fairy had institutions to care for the poor and sick of the district.[2]

By the 1850s the United Kingdom had a large number of charity hospitals for the sick poor, while the Poor Laws provided a nationwide "safety net" for the indigent. However, although charity hospitals were established in Victoria, the relative wealth of the colony compared with the British Isles meant that there was not the same pressure to set up a comprehensive system of poor relief. In Victoria in the nineteenth century for the most part wages were high and unemployment low; poverty was largely a problem of old age. As a result, the early charity hospitals had a dual role, that of treating the sick and caring for the aged poor. This dual role was reflected in the names of these institutions, which normally included the phrase, "hospital and benevolent asylum".

In the twentieth century, hospitals in the Western world became accepted as places of healing, where most diseases and injuries can be treated successfully. However, it is easy to forget that in 1850 medical science was in its infancy, with the first reported use of anaesthetics being in 1846, while Lister's work on antiseptics was over a decade away. Although doctors had developed elaborate classifications of diseases, they had little understanding of the causes of disease and many treatments were still based on folk medicine rather than science. Even the simplest abdominal surgery was considered impossible and a compound fracture normally resulted in amputation and frequently death. There were no effective treatments for diseases like diphtheria, typhoid, scarlet fever and tuberculosis, which were endemic and frequently fatal.[3]

The consequence of the limited knowledge of the causes of disease and infection was that hospitals in the mid-nineteenth century were very different from the twentieth century image of aseptic cleanliness. Since there was no understanding of germs, there was no awareness of the need for cleanliness. Hospitals were frequently filthy, surgeons operated wearing coats encrusted with blood from previous patients, and handwashing was rare. Consequently hospitals were centres of disease and infection and all who could afford to pay for medical attention would be cared for in their homes rather than in a hospital. There was a strong and not unjustified community perception that people only went to hospital to die.

Caring and efficient nurses are central to the image of the twentieth century hospital. Yet in 1850 Florence Nightingale had not yet begun her work which established the modern nursing profession and nursing in hospitals was largely the preserve of unskilled, untrained and unwashed men. Thus, when a group of philanthropic citizens of Warrnambool moved to establish a hospital in the town, the nature and purposes of this hospital were very different from those the institution developed in later years.

This is hinted at in a story in the *Portland Guardian* in September 1849, which told of a

> poor fellow named Partridge, who had been for some time ill in the district [and] came to Portland for medical aid. But he required nursing and bodily support, as well as medical attendance. [Rather than continuing to be a] burden of private individuals, he was assisted to proceed to Melbourne, but before he could obtain admission into the Hospital he died. Something should be done, on a small scale, by way of aiding persons in a similar destitute and painful condition.[4]

The most important purpose of the proposed hospital was to be an asylum for the destitute, while healing the sick was a secondary purpose, limited by the state of medical knowledge, which meant that those who could afford treatment at home had a far higher chance of recovery than those who had to seek treatment in a hospital.

The desire to replicate the institutions of civilisation was very strong in the pioneer settlements of the nineteenth century. Following its foundation in 1847, Warrnambool acquired a remarkable range of businesses and institutions in a very short time. By the early 1850s the new town had a newspaper, sporting and other clubs, churches, schools, several hotels, a wide variety of retailers, and a mechanics' institute. In this atmosphere it is not surprising that the citizens of Warrnambool felt the need to have a hospital for their community.

The first step toward the establishment of a hospital in Warrnambool is traditionally regarded as having occurred with the formation in June 1850 of a "Benevolent Committee" by "a few charitably disposed individuals."[5] A public meeting held on 18 June 1851 led to the establishment of the Warrnambool Benevolent Society, with the object of providing medical care and shelter for the needy. The early records of the Benevolent Society had disappeared before Richard Osburne wrote his history of Warrnambool in 1887 and we know very little of its activities. The first secretary of the society was Mr J. Pilkington, who was headmaster of the national school, but we do not know the foundation members of the committee of management. The first records of the committee date from 1853, when the Rev. James Dalrymple was chairman of a committee which included many of the leading citizens of early Warrnambool, such as Samuel Macgregor, J.M. Ardlie, James Cust, and William Bateman.

The most prominent figure on the early Benevolent Society committee was Richard Osburne, who succeeded Mr Pilkington as secretary in 1853 before serving as president from 1855 to 1861. Osburne was born in New South Wales in 1825 and served an apprenticeship as a printer on John Pascoe Fawkner's *Port Phillip Patriot* before coming to Warrnambool in 1847 as the correspondent for the *Argus* and several other newspapers and journals. In March 1851 he founded the *Warrnambool Examiner,* although, like most of the population of the town, he departed shortly afterwards for the goldfields, leaving the newspaper in recess until his return in 1853. Osburne played a prominent part in community affairs in Warrnambool and the Hospital, like the other institutions he supported, benefited greatly from the generous publicity he was able to give.

Rev. James Dalrymple was the first known chairman of the Benevolent Society, although he cannot have been the foundation chairman as he did not come to Warrnambool until 1853. Dalrymple was the second minister of the Presbyterian congregation in Warrnambool and Richard Osburne[6] described him as "a most eloquent preacher, and a useful public man in the town and district, taking a personal and active interest in the intellectual and religious improvement of the town." Most of the other known early committee members were local businessmen, lawyers, or government officials. It was very much a Warrnambool committee, with few, if any, members from the surrounding districts—a situation which can be explained by the difficulty of travelling to meetings.

Like many voluntary organisations, the Benevolent Society had to struggle with apathy among members of the committee and the wider community. The pages of the *Examiner* contained frequent complaints of lack of interest in the Hospital and pleas for greater involvement, particularly from country people. For example, in August 1858, Richard Osburne wrote:

> We really wish we could persuade some of our country friends to take even the slightest interest in the institution. We do not ask for money. Potatoes, firewood, anything in kind will be most thankfully received. The firewood consumed costs at least 15s per week, and a load brought into town now and then would not be a very great tax upon the farmers. Considering, also, that, at the lowest calculation, three-fourths of the cases relieved are from the country, common justice—if not humanity—demands that the country residents should take more interest than they do in the welfare of the Benevolent Asylum. The moment an individual is ill, he is brought into town, and in some cases actually left at the gates of the Asylum, but we regret to say, the treasurer cannot report that the subscriptions from the country are forwarded with the same celerity.[7]

Primarily as a means of enlisting greater support from country districts, in July 1855 the Warrnambool Hospital and Benevolent Asylum changed its name to the Villiers and Heytesbury Hospital and Benevolent Asylum.

In one of its earliest actions, the Benevolent Society petitioned the Government for a grant of land to build an asylum and in 1853 was given two acres in Ryot Street, part of the present Hospital site. In that year, the second annual meeting of the society showed receipts of £103 and expenditure of £15, leaving a credit balance of £87. At this stage the Benevolent Society had no buildings, no doctor and no paid staff. The society gave assistance to the destitute sick "by paying different parties to take the sick into their homes"; in the jargon of the day, "relief was administered outdoors". The number who received assistance in the first years of the Hospital is unclear, but it appears to have been very small. An article published in the *Examiner* by Richard Osburne in 1856 states that the number of patients cared for by the Benevolent Society had increased "twenty-fold" in the previous twelve months, and as the current number of patients on the books is given as seven, this increase obviously came off a very low base.[8]

This article is one of the few surviving documents from the earliest days of the Hospital and it deserves to be quoted at length as it does much to illustrate the early work of the Benevolent Society, and also clarifies several myths on the development of the Hospital:

> THE BENEVOLENT SOCIETY
>
> From the small amount of subscriptions received from the public, we may fairly assume for the sake of humanity, that it is not generally known that a society such as the above is in full working operation in the town of Warrnambool.
>
> The Warrnambool Benevolent Society was established in 1851, the object of that period being more to obtain the fines levied from the

drunkards at the Police Office, than from any urgent necessity then existing for its establishment. As the town increased, however, the great usefulness of such an institution was apparent to all and many a poor patient has had cause to bless its establishment.

During the last twelve months the number of patients have increased twenty fold in proportion to the number formerly on the books of the society, and in consequence of all the relief being administered out of doors, that is by paying different parties to take the sick into their homes and attend to them, the funds of the institution are now at a very low ebb indeed. The rates demanded, and in some instances paid, for attending to the sick have been most exorbitant, and the officers of the society were only warranted in paying such rates, by the laws of dire necessity. For when a poor wretch is dying, and £5 or £6 a week is demanded for attendance, the money is insignificant when placed in the balance with the life of a fellow creature.

Such have been some of the difficulties experienced by some of the officers of the Warrnambool Benevolent Society, and however much an ungrateful section of the community may grumble because things are not done in apple pie order, the former have the holy consolation of knowing that they have endeavoured to do their duty conscientiously, however thankless that duty may be.

As stated in a late number of this journal, the society have rented those premises formerly occupied by Dr Hutchinson, and have appointed a respectable married couple to take charge of the same. The premises are in a very healthy situation, and having a spacious garden attached thereto, are admirably adapted for the purpose. In consequence of the bedding etc, not yet being finished, a few days must yet elapse before the building will be ready for the reception of patients now on the books of the society, consisting of seven, for whom the large in aggregate, of upwards of £10 per week has been paid in the manner above stated by us.

In a short time the Society's patients will be under one roof, and the public will then have no excuse for not subsidising its wants. By the public we of course mean everyone, as we are aware that a few residents in the district have subscribed very handsomely to the funds of the Society. But we must reiterate that it is a disgrace to the public that so little has been subscribed to this institution. To the reapers, the splitters, the shearers, and those men who often pay the town a visit, we make an earnest appeal, on behalf of the Warrnambool Benevolent Society. Men of their class are generally the patients of the Society, men who have come down to the country to have a "spree", and who after their money goes, are left destitute and dying, until the Benevolent Society steps in and provides a comfortable asylum for them. To their comrades we appeal in particular, for we know they are as generous as they are reckless, and a few pounds from each will scarcely be missed, which in the aggregate would make up a large sum.

This article shows that the first actual hospital buildings were not occupied until April 1856, rather than 1854 as has often been stated.[9] These premises were on the corner of Koroit and Henna Streets, opposite Christ Church,

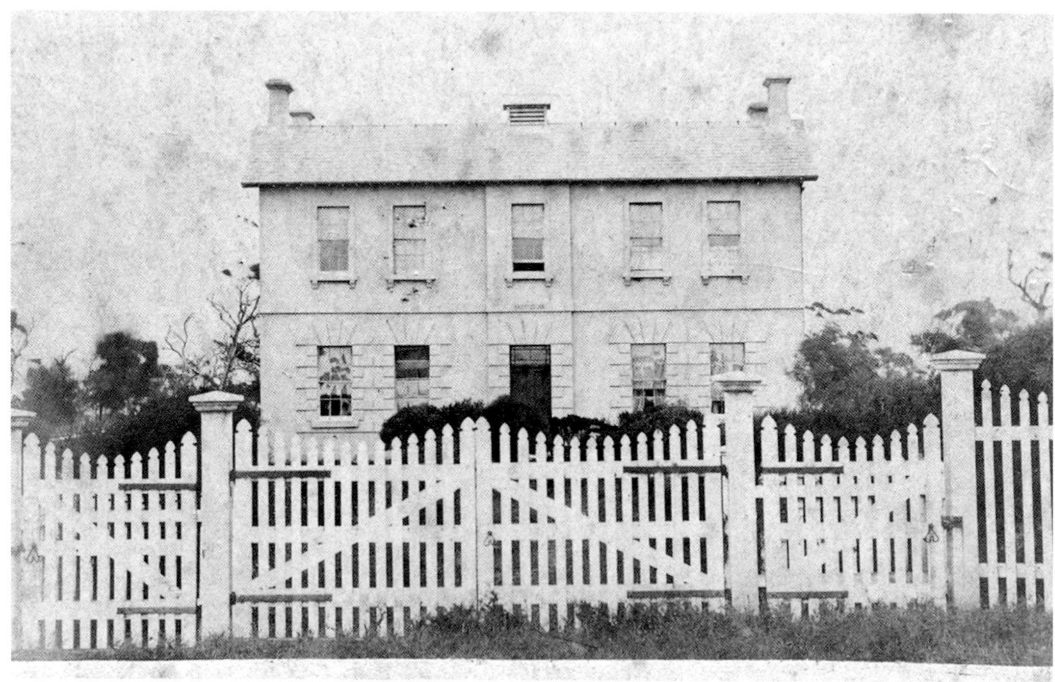

The Hospital area, 1861

and rented from Dr John Clarke, who took over the practice of Dr Hutchinson on the latter's retirement.[10] The "respectable married couple" who were appointed "master and matron" of the Hospital were Mr and Mrs J. Croll. Unfortunately we know nothing more about the woman who stands at the head of the Hospital's list of matrons and not even enough of Mr Croll's duties to say with any certainty whether he should be at the head of the list of chief executive officers or the list of janitors.

The first hospital had two wards, for male and female patients, apartments for the master and matron, a board room, "convenient out-offices" and a spacious yard and garden. In the first eight months the average number of patients in the Hospital was ten.[11]

Although we know very little of the patients cared for by the Benevolent Society in its early years, the article in the *Examiner* suggests that most were workers who had fallen on hard times, through age or the effects of alcohol. In the 1850s Victoria still had a large preponderance of males, and there were large numbers of single men with no family to fall back on in case of sickness or injury (or alcoholic stupor).[12] The Society devoted much of its efforts to the care of these men and it appealed (probably unavailingly) to men of the same class for financial assistance.

In the same month as the Benevolent Society opened the first hospital at the corner of Koroit and Henna Streets, the Government promised a substantial grant of £500 towards the construction of a more permanent building on the land already granted to the Society in Ryot Street, with the proviso that the local community raise an equivalent sum. For the next two years, the Society appears to have been too absorbed with the day to day running of its small hospital to devote much attention to building new premises. However, in October 1858 the *Examiner* reported that,

> Most strenuous efforts are at present being made to get up a sum of money in aid of the building fund of the Warrnambool Benevolent Asylum. . . The want of a building has long been felt, and we trust everyone will give a helping hand to further this desirable object.[13]

Over the years the Hospital has benefited from a wide variety of fundraising endeavours, and this tradition was established very early. The Benevolent Society organised a wide variety of fundraising events, from the traditional balls and concerts to the more unusual "Ethiopian entertainments" and performances by "Mr Testo, the Wizard". As Richard Osburne, the proprietor of the *Examiner*, was also the president of the Benevolent Society, the appeal for funds received strong support in that newspaper, with every donation to the building fund being acknowledged.

By 1860 the Society had raised sufficient funds to claim the Government grant and, in September 1860, contracts were let for the building of a hospital on the Ryot Street site. The building was designed by Andrew Kerr, the premier architect of early Warrnambool, and the largest contract, for the mason's work, was won by Jewell and Davidson. The building was finished by May 1861 and was "opened with all due formality".[14]

1 Rolf Boldrewood, *Old Melbourne Memories*, Melbourne, 1884, p.22.

2 The Port Fairy Hospital traces its origins back to 1846, thus predating the foundation of Warrnambool.

3 An excellent account of the development of medicine in the nineteenth century is in Richard Harrison Shryock, *The Development of Modern Medicine: An Interpretation of the Social and Scientific Factors Involved*, 3rd edn, Madison, Wisconsin, 1979.

4 *Portland Guardian*, 4 September 1849.

5 This story appears to have originated from Richard Osburne, who was probably a member of the inaugural committee; Richard Osburne, *The History of Warrnambool*, Melbourne, 1887, p.74.

6 Osburne, *History of Warrnambool*, p.42.

7 *Examiner*, 27 August 1858.

8 *Examiner*, 22 April 1856.

9 For example, C.E. Sayers and P.L. Yule, *By These We Flourish: A History of Warrnambool*, Warrnambool, 1987, p.161; Edward Vidler, *Warrnambool Past and Present*, Warrnambool, 1907, p.40.

10 *Examiner*, 11 April 1856.

11 *Examiner*, 17 February 1857.

12 For a discussion of the consequences of the preponderance of males in rural Victoria, see Margaret Kiddle, *Men of Yesterday: A Social History of the Western District of Victoria*, Melbourne, 1961, ch.4.

13 *Examiner*, 8 October 1858.

14 Osburne, *History of Warrnambool*, p.75.

Chapter 2

DOCTORS, NURSES, PATIENTS AND DISEASES

The history of the Warrnambool Base Hospital is intimately bound up with the story of the medical profession in the town. From the earliest days, the medical staff of the Hospital was made up of the town's doctors, with most of their service being honorary until the 1970s. In the nineteenth century, one of the doctors received a small payment as the Hospital's medical officer, with all other doctors being honoraries at the Hospital. This system continued until the practice of appointing recent graduates as resident medical officers began in 1902. From then until the increase in the number of specialists in Warrnambool from the 1970s, all patients at the Warrnambool Base Hospital were treated by one of the town's general practitioners, generally acting in an honorary capacity.

For the town's first one hundred years, there were remarkably few doctors in Warrnambool. A small number of long-serving doctors attended to the medical needs of the district's first four generations. Doctors such as Horace Holmes, Irving Buzzard, Egbert Connell, Thomas Fleetwood, Charles Macknight and Alf Brauer delivered babies, performed a wide range of surgery, gave anaesthetics and supervised the work of the resident doctors, as well as running large general practices.

In February 1849, when the settlement at Warrnambool was less than two years old, the correspondent of the *Portland Guardian* noted,

> There is neither a medical nor a legal gentleman residing within several miles of Warrnambool. The inhabitants especially to the former acquisition manifest some concern and appear desirous that a gentleman of that profession should be within reach in case of accident.[1]

The plea for a doctor for the town did not fall on deaf ears and by the end of 1849 two medical men had set up practices in the town. One of these was Dr Berkeley Hutchinson who practised from the house at the corner of Koroit and Henna Streets which later became the first hospital. The other was Dr Isaac Corney who set up a surgery and dispensary in a small wooden cottage in Banyan Street, near Merri Street. Dr Corney had studied medicine in London before joining his brothers on sheep runs in the Wando Vale and Casterton areas in the early 1840s. He died in 1854.

The surviving records suggest that as many as eleven other doctors may have practised in Warrnambool before 1860, although most of them stayed only a short time and had little or no impact on the development of the

Hospital.[2] Among the more prominent of these medical men, Dr Henry Thompson commenced practice in Merri Street in 1854. Dr Daniel Tierney was appointed public vaccinator [for smallpox] in 1855 and presumably also had a private practice. Dr Tierney was member of the Legislative Council for Western Province from 1856 to 1859 when he was disqualified "through not having sufficient amount of property."[3] Dr William Bainbridge practised in Warrnambool in 1858 and 1859. During this time he was criticised for negligence by a jury at an inquest and sued the well-known Anglican minister, Archdeacon Beamish, for non-payment of medical fees. He left Warrnambool in the early 1860s and died in Sale in 1876.[4] Dr Alexander Schultze is recorded as practising at Moloney's Woodford Inn in 1855, while the only record of Dr Husband is that he was in partnership with Dr John Clarke until he was killed in a fall from his horse at Wangoom in December 1856. Although it is likely that these doctors participated in the early work of the Benevolent Asylum, either by treating those eligible for "outdoor relief" or by honorary attendance to inpatients, their names are not mentioned in the few surviving records of the early days of the Hospital.

The two doctors who made the greatest contribution to the work of the Benevolent Society and the running of the Hospital in its earliest years were John Clarke and Henry Breton. John Clarke came to Warrnambool in 1852 and took over Dr Hutchinson's practice in 1854. He was probably the first medical officer for the Benevolent Society and was certainly the first medical officer to the Hospital when it opened next to his rooms in April 1856. Dr Clarke was also the council health officer and the coroner from 1855 to 1862. Initially his services to the Hospital were honorary, but at the annual meeting in 1859 it was resolved that he should be paid £50 annually. However, the following year, the subscribers to the Benevolent Society (who, as was the usual practice had the right to elect all officers, including medical staff), chose Dr Henry Breton ahead of Dr Clarke and then voted "that the thanks of the meeting be given to Dr Clarke for his past efficient services." No reasons were given for this abrupt dismissal, but it is more likely to have been a judgement of his personal popularity rather than a questioning of his professional capability. Little is known of his subsequent career; Richard Osburne states that he moved to Melbourne in 1862, although he again stood unsuccessfully for the position of paid medical officer in 1864.[5]

Dr Henry Breton is recorded as having been practising in Warrnambool by 1855. He was a graduate of Edinburgh University (at the time one of the world's leading medical schools) and had rooms in Gibson Street, next to the Customs office. In 1856 he succeeded Dr Tierney as "government doctor" in Warrnambool and is recorded as performing anaesthetics at the Hospital in 1858.[6] He only held the position of paid medical officer for two years, before being defeated in the election for the position by Dr R.H. Harrington.

It is difficult to assess the abilities and qualifications of Warrnambool's early medical practitioners. As there was no medical school in Australia until 1862, all these doctors had trained overseas, probably all in the United Kingdom. The first half of the nineteenth century was a period of rapid development in medical education in the United Kingdom, but the quality was still highly variable, ranging from the excellent training given at Edinburgh to the somewhat limited apprenticeship leading to an apothecaries certificate, which was nonetheless widely accepted as adequate for a general practitioner. The rapid rise in status of surgeons was only just beginning and a physician's qualification held far greater prestige than even membership of the Royal College of Surgeons.

The only readily accessible records of the qualifications of Warrnambool's early doctors are the claims made by doctors in newspaper advertisements, and in keeping with the ethics of the time it was probably those with the most doubtful qualifications who advertised the most. Dr Henry Thompson claimed to be a member of the Royal College of Surgeons, Dr Breton was a graduate of the University of Edinburgh, while Dr John Clarke claimed to be both a doctor of medicine and a member of the Royal College of Surgeons and Alexander Schultze was an M.D. and "formerly President of the Royal Medical Society of Edinburgh". Legal regulation of the medical profession in Victoria was less than rigorous in this period and the range of qualifications and abilities of Warrnambool's early doctors was probably highly variable.

The mid-nineteenth century was a period of revolutionary progress in the development of modern medicine. The introduction of anaesthesia in the 1840s, the work of Pasteur in demonstrating the "germ theory of disease causation", coupled with Lister's practical extension of this theory to show that wound infection could be controlled, transformed surgery from "an ancient but very limited art . . . into a potent and impressive science".[7] From the early 1860s Pasteur's work led to the development of bacteriology and the demonstration that bacteria cause diseases, with the subsequent development of vaccines and anti-toxins for several of the most common diseases. At a more immediately practical level, Lister showed the importance of cleanliness, and hospitals were quickly transformed from centres of infection into the spotlessly white, aseptic institutions they are today. Progress in science transformed hospitals from places where the destitute went to die, to places of healing.

In 1847 Warrnambool was among the newest and most remote outposts of Western civilisation, and even in the 1860s it was still extremely isolated, with no railway, poor roads and an expensive and dangerous sea passage the main means of travel to Melbourne. The sea voyage from Europe to Australia was still measured in months rather than weeks. Although there is very little evidence, it appears that the new discoveries in medicine were adopted fairly quickly by Warrnambool doctors. For example, the following report indicates a routine use of anaesthesia in surgery by 1858:

A poor fellow named Kendall, formerly a hawker in this district, and who has been an inmate of the Hospital for the past nine months, suffering under a compound fracture of the leg, underwent an operation last week. His leg was amputated below the knee most successfully by Dr. Clarke, assisted by Dr. Breton, and Dr. Boyd, of Belfast. The operation was performed whilst the patient was under the influence of chloroform, which was administered by Dr. Breton.[8]

Other evidence suggests that for most conditions the treatments given to patients in the Hospital were very basic. In October 1859 Dr Clarke reported that many recent cases "were of a very distressing character, requiring in every instance extra diet, together with a more than usual quantity of stimuli".[9] While modern medicine agrees on the importance of diet, the widespread use of "stimuli" (meaning alcohol) declined rapidly in the late ninteenth century. However, in the 1850s alcohol was widely prescribed as a medicine, even for very young babies, and it is probable that the Warrnambool Hospital spent more on wine and spirits than on all other medicines put together.

There are only a few brief reports which give us an insight into the lives of the patients who were cared for by the Warrnambool Hospital in the 1850s. Again, it is necessary to remember that the most important role of the Hospital in its earliest years was "to relieve the destitute of the district".[10] Healing the sick was a secondary aim, largely because the current state of medical knowledge meant that for most conditions little could be done. While the Benevolent Society was based in rented premises, the number of patients treated was very small, and the time they each stayed in the Hospital was very long. In May 1856 the managing committee reported "There are at present six male patients on the premises, and there will be a female, as soon as the female ward is completed."[11] Three years later the society's annual report stated,

The number of patients admitted into the Asylum during the year has been 32, of whom 7 have died, 12 have been discharged cured, 3 have been forwarded to Melbourne, and 10 are at present inmates of the Asylum. The number of persons who have received out door relief for various periods has been 5.[12]

The death rate of over twenty per cent reflects the facts that a majority of patients were elderly and that there were very few useful treatments available for most medical conditions. It is unfortunate that we do not know more about the three patients who were forwarded to Melbourne. Were these serious cases going to Melbourne specialists or simply cases of destitution being sent to the Benevolent Hospital in the city or even to jobs?

In July 1856, the *Examiner* published a story which illustrates the inability of doctors to treat many common conditions:

DEATH IN THE HOSPITAL

On Saturday last, a young man, named James Carpenter, a blacksmith, in the employ of Mr Foote, Timor Street, was admitted into the Hospital, but died a few hours afterward. It appears that he had been suffering very severely for the past few weeks from diarrhoea, and his friends thought he would be much better attended to in the Hospital whence he was admitted on a certificate from his medical attendant. Deceased was a native of Tasmania, and was about twenty years of age.[13]

The first surviving record of the diseases treated at the Warrnambool Hospital is that published in the annual report for 1860.[14] While the total number of patients (fifty-one) was too small to be statistically significant, it nonetheless gives some indication of the more common diseases treated. The most common problem was abscesses, understandable in an era when the cause of infection was not understood and there was no means of controlling it. Four patients with dyspepsia were successfully treated, but one of the four victims of influenza died in the Hospital. Delirium tremens was given as the cause of admission for three patients, chronic conjunctivitis and rheumatism for two each, while all the other ailments ranging from amolissement of the brain and snake bite to debility and burns had only single admissions. It is surprising that there was only one patient admitted with phthisis (tuberculosis), as this is generally regarded as having been endemic in the mid-nineteenth century. Similarly surprising is the absence of patients with gastroenteritis, enteric fever, typhoid or any of the other disorders of the gastrointestinal tract common in the days of impure food, uncertain water supply, poor drainage and, especially, no adequate means of sewerage disposal. These diseases, which were not fully differentiated until the last decades of the century, were widespread in Victorian towns before 1900, particularly in summer. The 1860 annual report also makes the first mention of the treatment of Aboriginal patients, with three being treated as inpatients and another receiving outdoor relief.

The day to day care of the patients in the Hospital was in the hands of the master and matron, positions which were normally held by a married couple. Mr and Mrs Croll remained until early 1859, when Mr and Mrs Mainwaring were appointed at a combined salary of £100 with board and residence. Mr Mainwaring's previous position was a wardsman in the Melbourne Hospital, in the period when many of the tasks which later came to be performed by female nurses, were carried out primarily by male wardsmen. The Crolls and the Mainwarings were regularly commended in the medical officer's reports to the committee of management for the cleanliness of the Hospital and the excellent care they gave the patients. There is no surviving record of other staff employed at the Hospital in the 1850s. It is uncertain whether the Hospital had any cooks, gardeners, cleaners or other staff, or whether the master and matron carried out these tasks in addition to their role in patient care.

By the time the new Hospital opened in Ryot Street in 1861, the Villiers and Heytesbury Hospital and Benevolent Asylum was a well established Warrnambool institution. It provided the main social security for the aged, infirm and destitute of the town and district. The poor had become accustomed to relying on it for first aid treatment of injuries, though possibly less so for disease unless forced by lack of alternative care. The doctors of the town had begun their long tradition of honorary service to the Hospital, and the first matrons had begun the tradition of skilled and caring nursing. For the people of the town, the Hospital had become one of the main focuses for charitable work and, after initial resistance, the people of the district were beginning to support the institution. With the opening of the new Hospital, the increasing pace of improvement in medical knowledge and the beginnings of the nursing profession, the 1860s marked the start of a period of solid growth for Warrnambool Hospital.

[1] *Portland Guardian*, 12 February 1849.
[2] Unpublished list of early doctors of south-west Victoria compiled by Stephen C. Due, medical librarian, Geelong Hospital, December 2000.
[3] Osburne, *History of Warrnambool*, p.183.
[4] Warrnambool and District Historical Society, *Newsletter*, February 2001, p.3.
[5] Osburne, *History of Warrnambool*, p.68.
[6] *Examiner*, 3 December 1858.
[7] Shryock, *Development of Modern Medicine*, p.281.
[8] *Examiner*, 3 December 1858.
[9] *Examiner*, 14 October 1859.
[10] *Examiner*, 3 June 1859.
[11] *Examiner*, 6 May 1856.
[12] *Examiner*, 18 February 1859.
[13] *Examiner*, 8 July 1856.
[14] *Examiner*, 1 February 1861.

Chapter 3

COMMITTEE, BUILDINGS AND FINANCES, 1861–1900

Following the opening of the new premises in May 1861, the Warrnambool Hospital entered a long period of steady growth. Over the next forty years the number of patients continued to increase, the Hospital obtained more land and more buildings, its income and expenditure increased by more than four times and both its medical and non-medical staff increased proportionately.

The committee of the Hospital in this period remained exclusively male, overwhelmingly Protestant and socially homogenous. The members came from the town's commercial and professional elite, together with some representation from squatters and larger farmers in the surrounding district. The committee worked unobtrusively but very effectively to advance the interests of the Hospital and provide care for the sick, injured and destitute of the district.

The archetypal Hospital committee member of the nineteenth century was Frederick Stevens, who served on the committee from 1859 to 1872, being president and treasurer for most of this time. Stevens was born in 1821, being a general merchant in Melbourne and then Belfast before coming to Warrnambool in the mid-1850s. He went into partnership in Timor Street with Thomas Denney and appears to have been highly successful, being a director of many local companies. A wide range of community groups benefited from Frederick Stevens' involvement and generosity. In addition to his commitment to the Hospital, he was president of the Horticultural Society, vice-chairman of the Walter Scott centenary committee, and a strong supporter of the Framlingham Aboriginal community. In common with most Hospital committee members, Stevens was a Protestant, being a leading member of the Christ Church congregation. There was no tokenism in Frederick Stevens' commitment to these organisations; he rarely missed a Hospital committee meeting over the period of his membership.

Those who followed Frederick Stevens in the presidency of the Hospital were in the same mould. Charles Cramer (president 1872–75) was a successful businessman and served two terms as mayor, before becoming town clerk in 1877. He was succeeded by J.G. Cramond, co-founder of Cramond and Dickson's, followed in turn by Thomas King, one of the town's longest serving councillors. The presidents were very much a reflection of the overall structure of the committee.

From 1871 the committee was made up of town and country members, to reflect the Hospital's role in providing care for the sick, injured and destitute from the town of Warrnambool and its surrounding district and the support given to the Hospital by the town and shire councils. The social background of the country members appears to have been slightly broader than that of the town members. For example, the country members of the committee elected in January 1873 included pastoralists such as James Glowery of Yalloak, John Thomson of Keilambete,[1] Robert Hood of Merrang and Thomas Shaw of Darlington, as well as Patrick Conrick, a Catholic farmer of Yangery, Charles Norman, a Koroit shopkeeper, William Halliwell, who had a dairy farm at Cudgee and J.M. Patison, the postmaster at Woodford.

The role of the members of the committee was not limited to making up the numbers at meetings; they were expected to, and did, take an active part in many aspects of the running of the Hospital. The most important of these was probably fundraising, but there was also a regular roster for the committee members to make tours of inspection of the Hospital, and they generally appear to have been diligent in carrying out this task.

Less is known of most who served as secretaries to the committee over this period. Initially this was an honorary position, held by one of the gentlemen of the committee, but from 1859 it became a salaried position. The first paid secretary was Mr John Mainwaring, who held the position

Warrnambool Hospital c.1910

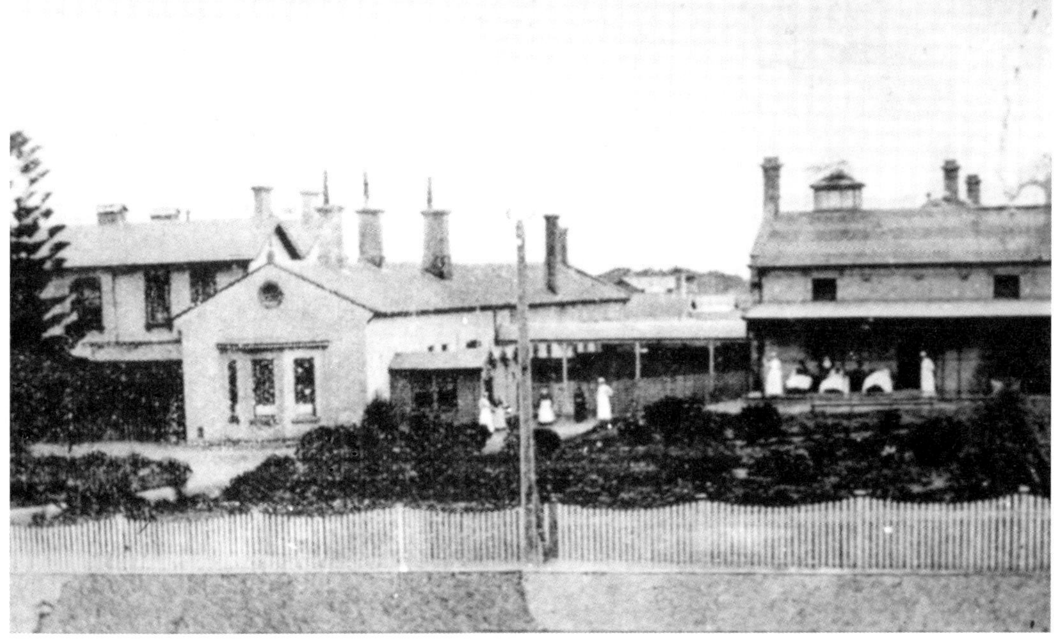

concurrent with his role as master—unfortunately no job description has survived, so we do not know what was expected of him.[2] Following the departure of Mr and Mrs Mainwaring, Alfred Davies became secretary. Davies was secretary to the Shire of Warrnambool and a prominent figure in local government in the district, so his role as hospital secretary must have been a very part time job. He retained the position until 1877, when he mysteriously disappeared at the same time as his close friend, Henry Read, the Warrnambool borough clerk. Investigations showed that Read had misappropriated large sums from the Warrnambool Building Society, and small sums were missing from the Warrnambool Cemetery Trust and the Warrnambool Shire for which Davies was responsible. No money was missing from the Hospital accounts, but the committee had to seek a new secretary as Davies was never heard of again in the district.[3] The new secretary was John Cleverdon, an accountant and auditor, who was prominent in local affairs. Cleverdon held the position until 1897, when he apparently became insane and was incarcerated in the Kew Mental Hospital.

The increasing demands on the services of the Hospital led to a steady expansion of buildings and facilities throughout the latter decades of the nineteenth century. The first major task following the opening of the first building in Ryot Street in 1861 was to complete fencing and laying out the grounds. In May of that year the committee called for tenders for "grubbing and clearing" five acres, reflecting the fact that the site granted to the Benevolent Society was still uncleared bush on the edge of Warrnambool. Over the next few years the Hospital's land was cleared and turned into an efficient small farm to provide fresh produce for the patients and staff. By the mid-1870s the Hospital had a dairy, a piggery and a highly productive vegetable patch. In addition to providing fresh produce for the Hospital, it is probable that the Hospital's farming activities were an early form of occupational therapy. Many of the Hospital's long term patients were destitute rather than seriously ill, and it seems likely that they were largely responsible for caring for the cows, pigs and vegetable patch.

The number of patients doubled within eight years of the opening of the new hospital and, by the late 1860s, the steady increase in demand led the committee to plan for extensions. From 1866 the committee began to call for government assistance to construct a fever ward in which to treat patients with infectious diseases. This is an interesting reflection of the growing awareness of the ways in which diseases are transmitted and the dangers of having infectious patients in general wards with other patients. However, the Hospital committee appears to have been ahead of the Government in this and no government assistance was forthcoming until 1878.

Although the Government did not fund a fever ward of the size envisaged by the Hospital committee, it did make a grant of £400, which, with the addition of local contributions, enabled the committee to proceed with a

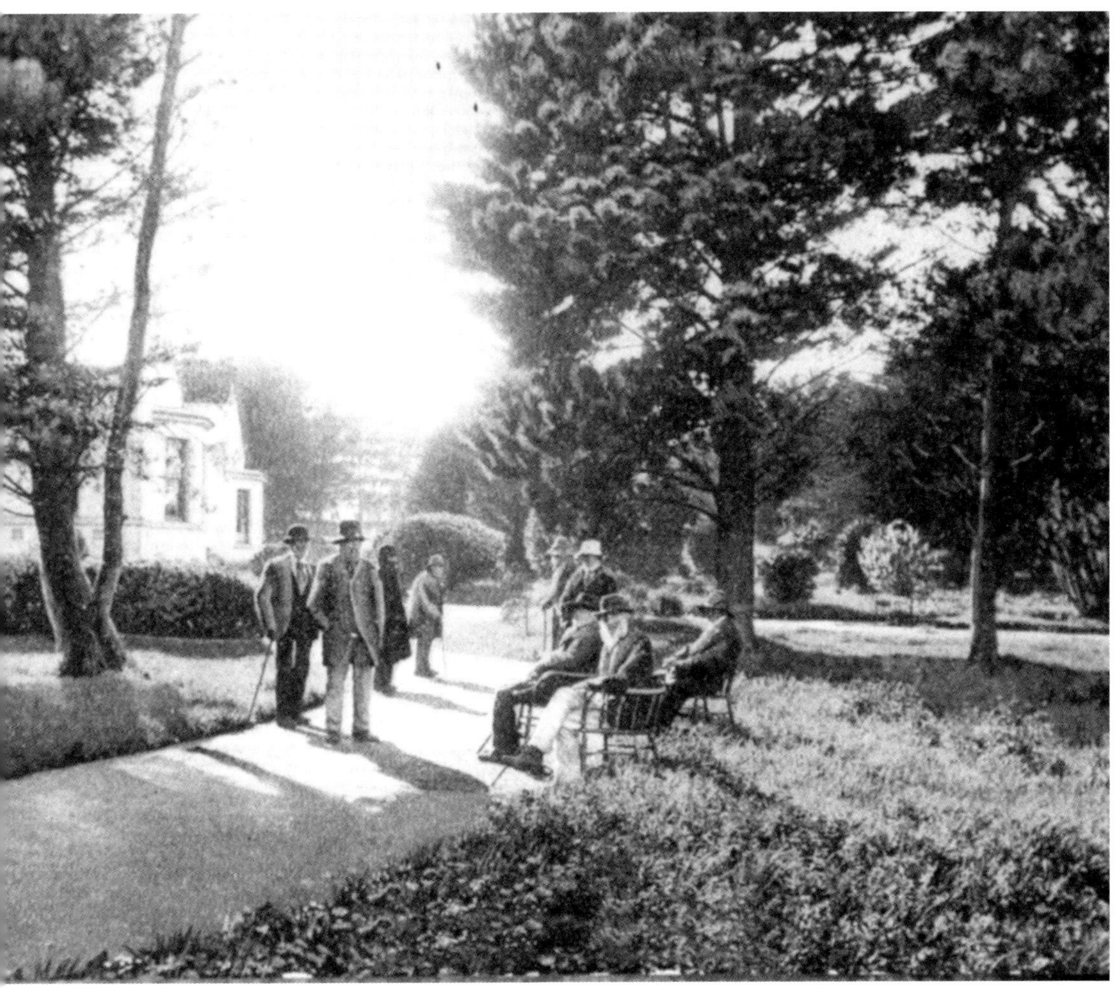

Patients in the Hospital grounds c.1900

substantial expansion project, doubling the size of the Hospital. By 1870 the Hospital had "a fever ward, female ward, two male wards, dining room, board room, operating room and staff rooms" and it could accommodate twenty-seven male and nine female patients.[4] The disparity in numbers between males and females is a reflection of the fact that, although Victorian society was stabilising after the pioneering days and the goldrushes, there was still a large preponderance of men among older age groups.

In this period the committee frequently undertook minor works. For example, in January 1873 the annual report noted that the previous year had seen "the laying out and planting of the grounds, the construction of a hot water bath, further drainage of the yard, and enlargement and paving of the piggeries".[5]

During the 1870s there was a steady decline in the levels of public health in Warrnambool. The town was not alone in this—a result of the pressure of increasing population on inadequate drainage, sewerage and

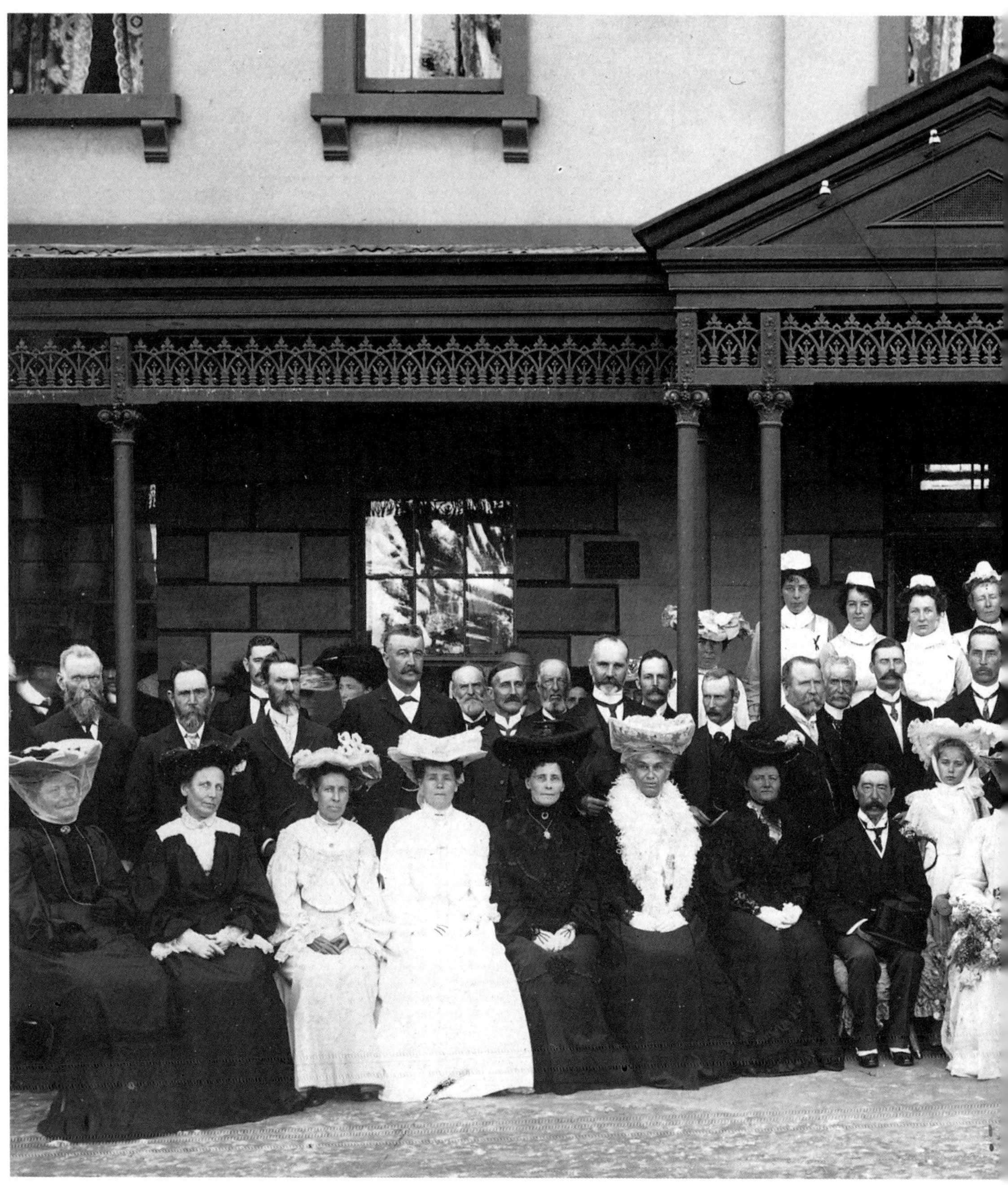

water supply, combined with an increase in the number of infectious diseases prevalent in Australia. This latter phenomenon saw many of the endemic diseases of Europe such as diphtheria, scarlet fever, typhoid and others appear in Australia for the first time in the mid-nineteenth century and spread rapidly among a population with lower resistance than most European populations.[6] Typhoid in particular became a major cause of

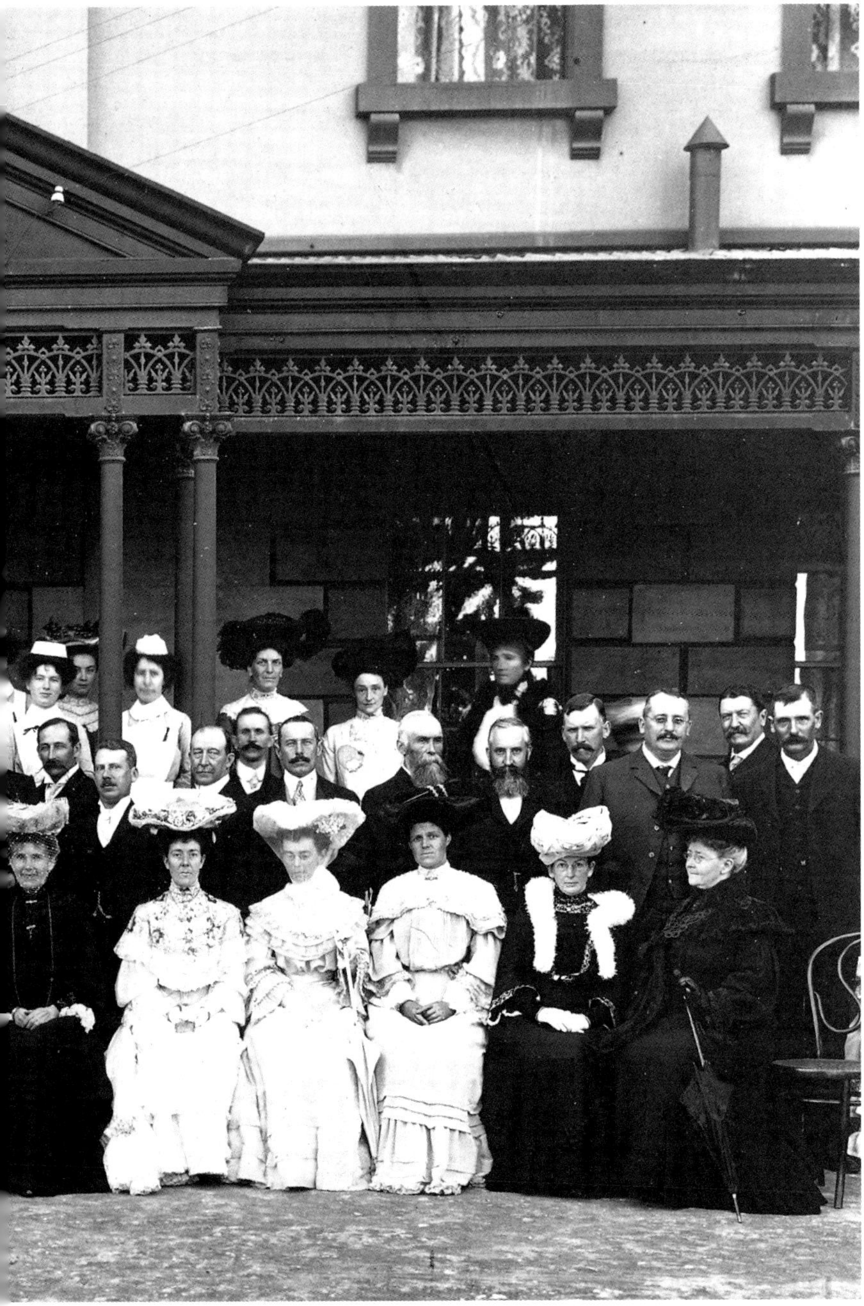

Lord and Lady Northcote and others at Warrnambool Hospital, 1905.

morbidity and mortality, with epidemics occurring almost every summer, while diphtheria, scarlet fever, whooping cough and "summer diarrhoea" were major causes of the very high child mortality of the period.

Although it was many years before the necessary preventive measures such as a clean water supply and sewerage were provided in Warrnambool, the Hospital committee collaborated with the borough and shire councils and the Public Health Department to provide an infectious diseases ward for the district. This prison-like ward was built in the Hospital grounds in 1878. Initially its maintenance was the responsibility of the borough and shire councils, but from 1882 the committee took over the running of the ward, with financial support from the two councils. The committee also tried to ensure a pure water supply for the Hospital by sinking a well in the grounds.

During the 1880s, as the population grew and the number of old people in the colony expanded, the facilities of the Hospital were placed under increasing pressure. An article in the *Standard* in 1886 summarised the situation:

> The patching which is continually being executed in connection with the Hospital and Benevolent Asylum is evidence of the inadequacy of that building for the purposes it is designed to fulfil. At times a ward is added here, a room there, and some convenience somewhere else, but it still remains a patchwork building, not at all adapted for the purposes of an Hospital. The recent additions to the main structure, [new kitchens] though in every way required . . . are simply an excrescence jutting out at the rear, and calculated to decrease the purity of the air within the main building . . . Another matter of complaint is the ventilation of the building, and the extremely awkward condition of the female benevolents and hospital patients who occupy the upper floor of the main building. The house, moreover, is always inconveniently crowded, beds having to be made up for patients on the floor . . . the building, as a hospital, is defective from floor to ceiling, and from the front entrance to the back.[7]

The article continued to argue that the time was approaching when the two functions of the Hospital—as a hospital for the sick and as a benevolent asylum for the aged poor—should be separated and a completely new hospital building should be built. However, although there was considerable support for this proposition, it was not financially feasible at that time, so the Hospital committee devoted considerable effort to renovating and rebuilding the existing facilities.

In 1886 the Hospital committee decided to alter the exclusively benevolent character of the institution by admitting paying patients for the first time. Two bedrooms and a sitting room were provided for paying patients, but there is little information as to the extent of their use or the revenue gained. It seems probable that most people who could afford to pay for medical treatment chose to go to one of the town's private hospitals rather than be associated with a benevolent institution for the poor.

During 1889 the committee built a new wing to provide eighteen new beds, giving a total of sixty-eight beds, thirty for hospital patients and thirty-eight for the "aged, poor and decrepit", and two years later a new female ward was opened on the ground floor. However, the onset of the depression of the 1890s prevented further extensions for the rest of the decade, even though the harsh economic times meant that the demands on the Hospital were greater than ever. The one exception was a major refit for the fever ward, which was financed by the Warrnambool town and shire councils in 1898.

It is difficult to give a picture of the Warrnambool Hospital in the last decades of the nineteenth century. Few drawings or plans survive, so we must rely largely on the few available descriptions. The Hospital was far from the modern image of a hospital, but it was also unlike the general picture of a late nineteenth century hospital, typified for Victorians by Melbourne's old Queen Victoria Hospital in Lonsdale Street or the old Children's Hospital in Carlton, with their ornate, red brick pavilions, and large, high ceilinged wards with up to fifty beds. The Warrnambool Hospital by 1900 was an unplanned straggle of buildings set among landscaped gardens. The buildings were of the same style and size as shops and houses in Warrnambool and the Hospital was not architecturally differentiated from the rest of the community as it has inevitably become today. Perhaps we could liken it to a small village with its houses, cottages and gardens.

Although the scale of operations of the Warrnambool Hospital increased substantially between 1860 and 1900, the sources of income and the proportion of income derived from each changed substantially. In the 1860s and 1870s, over half the Hospital's income came from the government grant, with the rest being raised locally. In 1873, the Hospital's income of £919 was made up of government grants of £578, subscriptions and donations of £292, patient payments of £1/8/9 and proceeds from sale of vegetables and livestock of £34. Although the Hospital's expenditure rose steeply over the last quarter of the century, the government grant did not rise at all and the committee was forced to look to the local community for a far higher proportion of its income.

The most consistent form of continuing fundraising was through subscriptions. Subscribers to the Hospital played a more important role than just providing funds, being, in fact, the ultimate governing body of the institution, electing the committee and medical officers. From 1861 the Hospital had a by-law that patients could only be admitted on the written recommendation of a subscriber. A sliding scale was introduced to encourage higher subscriptions—subscribers of one guinea (£1/1/-) could recommend one patient annually, subscribers of three guineas, two patients, five guineas, three patients and so on. This rule was enforced except in cases of emergency and remained in place until 1928. A majority of the leading citizens of the town and district were subscribers.

The Hospital has always been able to enlist the support of the whole community for major fundraising efforts. The building projects of 1861 and 1869 were largely financed by enormous bazaars which raised hundreds of pounds. The *Examiner* reported on the first of these:

> The Fancy Bazaar in aid of the Benevolent Asylum was concluded on Saturday night, and we are sure the ladies and gentlemen who undertook the management of the same, must have been heartily pleased when all was over. For months previous the utmost energies of those who were

working for the Bazaar had been taxed to the utmost, and although the wonderful success which was attained must have been some solace for the self-sacrifice, yet we are certain everyone was glad when the Bazaar was closed. The result exceeded all expectation. It was expected that about £400 would be realised, but although the actual amount was not known in time for this day's paper, it is anticipated the total amount taken during the past three days will amount to £700 at the least.

> We had intended to comment on each stall and each particular article of merit, but really we would be pushed for room even if we had a daily paper. All the stalls were good and well attended to, and if in our small but spirited community we might be permitted to make an exception, let it be in favour of those ladies who undertook the refreshment stall. Every lady in the Bazaar had hard work to do, and most nobly did they attend to their duties. Such an example of self-denial and generosity has seldom been seen . . .We have nothing but praise for the work of the ladies of the Warrnambool district in the holy and blessed cause of charity and we can say truly that they have done so disinterestedly and may they meet their due reward hereafter.[8]

From the late 1870s, the Hospital's funds received a very welcome annual boost from Hospital Saturday and Hospital Sunday. On the former day, hospitals and benevolent asylums held open days and raised funds from small admission fees and donations, while on the latter, hospitals received the proceeds of church collections. These special days raised substantial amounts. In 1887, for example, Hospital Saturday and Hospital Sunday raised £331 of the Hospital's total income of £1486.[9]

The Warrnambool Hospital also benefited from innumerable smaller fundraising activities. These ranged from "soirees" and concerts to donations of firewood, fruit, and vegetables. Soirees were a combination of amateur entertainment and supper, popular in the 1850s and 1860s. In December 1859 the *Examiner* gave a very full account of a soiree held by the Yangery Mutual Improvement Society in aid of the Hospital. The soiree was held in the Midgley's barn at Yangery Grange and after a "bountiful repast", those attending were treated to lectures on subjects including "The Moral Condition of the Colony", and "The Cultivation of Reason", a selection of songs and a piano programme performed by Miss Macdonald of Warrnambool.[10]

Many concerts, sporting events, dances and other functions were held to benefit the Hospital's finances, and these were generally well supported by the public. One regular fundraising event in the 1880s was the annual "drum-head" service. The 1887 service was typical:

> The drum-head service in aid of the funds of the Warrnambool Hospital was held yesterday in the Hospital grounds. The unpleasant heat of the weather deterred a great many from attending. About four hundred people assembled on the ground. The Militia marched to the scene of the proceedings accompanied by the band, and after the conclusion of the service marched back to the Orderly Room. The music by the choir and the

band formed a very attractive feature of the service. The Ven. Archdeacon Beamish presided, and gave the Scripture reading, prayer was offered by the Rev. R. Keith Mackay, and an effective sermon was delivered by the Rev. Geo. Tait. The proceeds of the collection amounted to £15 14s 7d.[11]

In a period when the greater part of funds had to be raised locally, the Hospital enjoyed consistent support from the people of the town. In the first two decades of the Hospital's existence, the committee frequently complained of the paucity of support from the surrounding districts, but this was gradually remedied and by the 1880s the Hospital was well supported by the region—roughly definable at this time as the area within a day's return travel.

[1] John Thomson was one of the Warrnambool Hospital's most generous benefactors, leaving the Hospital about £12,000 on his death in 1890.
[2] Richard Osburne stated that James Hider was the first paid secretary (*History of Warrnambool*, p.76), but it appears likely that Hider was actually the last of the honorary secretaries or else was secretary to the committee (of which he was a member) rather than the Benevolent Society. All reports between 1859 and 1862 name Mr J. Mainwaring as secretary.
[3] C.E. Sayers, *Of Many Things: A History of Warrnambool Shire*, Melbourne, 1972, pp.62–64.
[4] Quoted in *Warrnambool Standard*, 22 March 1947.
[5] *Standard*, 10 January 1873.
[6] This phenomenon is discussed in Bryan Gandevia, *Tears Often Shed: Child Health and Welfare in Australia from 1788*, Sydney, 1978, p.36.
[7] *Standard*, 8 December 1886.
[8] *Examiner*, 1 January 1861.
[9] *Standard*, 8 January 1888.
[10] *Examiner*, 13 December, 1859.
[11] *Standard*, 10 January 1887.

Chapter 4

DOCTORS AND DISEASES

"The influence of living organisms . . . in the production of diseased conditions in man . . . has excited much attention in the last few years."[1] With these words, Dr James Jamieson began the most important contribution to medical literature by a Warrnambool doctor. "On the Parasitic Theory of Disease" was not an article based on original research (although Jamieson referred frequently to his own observations over the years) but was a masterly summary of the work of Pasteur, Lister and other leading British and European bacteriologists, biologists and medical scientists, put in a form which was accessible to the Victorian medical profession. This article was highly influential at the time and effectively ended the local controversy between supporters and opponents of the idea that bacteria cause disease, with the latter group being effectively silenced.

The controversy over the causes of disease might seem almost quaint today, but at the time it was hard fought and had great practical significance for the treatment of patients. The need for Dr Jamieson's powerful article is reflected in a paper, typical of many others, published in 1868. Dr John Day of Geelong, writing on diphtheria argued that that disease was "caused by the presence in the atmosphere of some highly oxidising substance, probably ozone".[2] Dr Day went on to refer approvingly to a theory that "certain diseases, such as Whooping Cough, Measles, Scarlatina and Cholera [were] in some way under the influence of Terrestrial Magnetism [and] that Magnetic Storms may be intimately concerned in the causation of certain epidemic diseases." From this Dr Day deduced that the best form of treatment was to move the patient away from the magnetic disturbance! Convincing the medical profession of the validity of the germ theory of disease was an essential preliminary to pursuing rational and effective forms of treatment. This was clearly appreciated at the time; as Dr Jamieson wrote,

> A rational treatment of any disease must always be dependent on a knowledge of its causation; and so long as we are in the dark about the agents or influences which originate or keep up diseased conditions, our efforts in the way of prevention and cure, however apparently successful, must always bear the taint of uncertainty.[3]

From this he argued that an acceptance of the germ theory of disease would lead people to see the need for hygiene and encourage the "free and careful use of those agents known as disinfectants".

The theoretical innovations of Pasteur and Lister and their practical application formed the basis of both medical and surgical practice until the development of antibiotics in the 1940s. Dr Jamieson discussed many of these applications in his article: antiseptic surgery, the prevention of puerperal fever, and the cure of erysipelas and related diseases, which were largely the product of poor hygiene in hospitals. Jamieson also looked forward to the time when doctors could [4]attack diseases in the body, rather than just on the skin, speculating on the possibility of using "disinfectants as internal remedies." Jamieson did not anticipate other innovations which developed from the new science of bacteriology, in particular the invention of vaccines and anti-toxins, but his hopes for the future of medicine were such that he would not have been surprised by these developments.

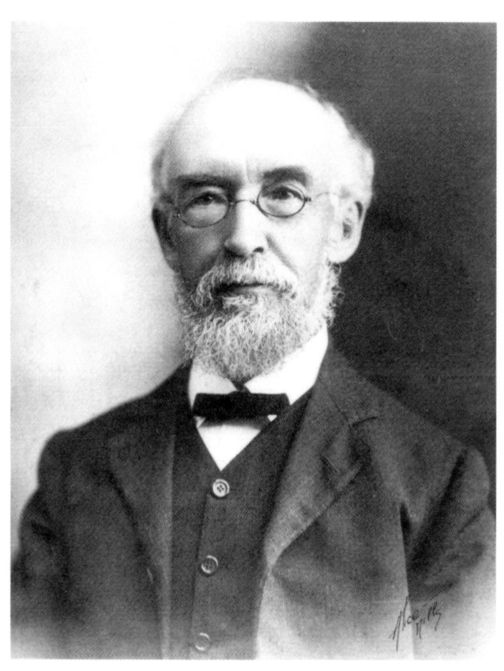

Dr James Jamieson

Dr James Jamieson had studied medicine at Glasgow University, where he graduated as doctor of medicine in 1862 and master of surgery in 1863. At Glasgow Jamieson was almost certainly a student of Lister, who became Professor of Surgery there in 1860, although his seminal work on antiseptic surgery was not published until 1867. In 1864 Jamieson migrated to Australia, coming to Warrnambool where his brother (after whom Jamieson Street is named) was a prominent businessman and councillor. In his thirteen years in Warrnambool Dr Jamieson built up a successful private practice, and served the Hospital as an honorary medical officer, as well as participating actively in medical politics and controversies in Melbourne. He eventually moved to Melbourne in 1877 where he went on to a highly distinguished career as Professor of Medicine at the University of Melbourne, honorary physician to the Alfred Hospital, editor of the *Australian Medical Journal* and Health Officer to the City of Melbourne.[5]

It is difficult to assess the extent to which the advanced ideas of Dr Jamieson affected the practice of medicine in Warrnambool, but it seems likely that he would have insisted on modern standards of cleanliness and hygiene in the Hospital and encouraged the early use of Listerian methods in surgery.

While James Jamieson was the most academically distinguished doctor to practice in Warrnambool in the nineteenth century, the other doctors included some notable medical men as well as a solid group of dedicated general practitioners. One of the most extraordinary characters ever to serve on the honorary staff of the Warrnambool Hospital was John Singleton. Dr Singleton trained in Ireland and practised in Melbourne in the 1850s before moving to Warrnambool in 1860. In his memoirs, Singleton described Warrnambool as

> a beautifully situated seaport in the western district, within twelve or fifteen hours by steamboat, or a day by coach and train of Melbourne . . . The district is a farming one—the richest probably in the colony . . . But I found drunkenness abounding to a frightful extent, producing accidents, suicides, insanity and disease, and causing the majority of the deaths that occurred among the adult population. Ignorance prevailed, and such amusements as racing and others of a similar character, led to habits of dissipation in town and country; and among every class the same degrading and ruinous habits prevailed.[6]

Singleton built up an extensive practice in Warrnambool and the surrounding district and involved himself deeply in "good works", notably the temperance campaign and care of the local Aboriginal population. He served on the honorary staff of Warrnambool Hospital and in 1864 he wrote to the Hospital committee "offering his services gratis to the Institution for three or four months, and trusting the other medical gentlemen would similarly give their services during the remainder of the year."[7] However, the committee felt that the interests of patients would be best served by having a permanent, paid medical officer at the Hospital.

While John Singleton was noted as one of Victoria's great philanthropists and temperance campaigners until his death in 1891—being a founder of the Royal Children's Hospital and other community medical services in inner Melbourne which are still in existence—not all of Warrnambool's medical practitioners followed his example. Joseph Mackenzie held the prestigious appointment of senior resident medical officer at the Melbourne Hospital before commencing practice in Koroit Street in 1870. However, his career was not a success and he died an alcoholic in 1872. His obituary in the *Australian Medical Journal* was a masterpiece of brevity:

> Dr Mackenzie had good abilities and excellent opportunities. He failed to use the former and he wasted the latter. His life and death are alike warnings.[8]

Most Warrnambool doctors lacked the public profile of Drs Jamieson and Singleton and the notoriety of Dr Mackenzie. Drs William Boyd, Thomas Embling, William Loftus, Frederick Moreton, Thomas Fleetwood, Lindsay Miller and others gave years of dedicated service to Warrnambool Hospital and the community. The central medical figure in the development of the Hospital in the 1860s, 70s and 80s was Dr R.H. Harrington, who was the medical officer from 1862 until his retirement in 1889. Unfortunately we know relatively little about Dr Harrington. He trained in Britain, becoming a member of the Royal College of Physicians, and arrived in Warrnambool in about 1860. In January 1862 he stood against Dr Breton for the position of paid medical officer to the Warrnambool Hospital and won a clear victory, receiving thirty-five votes from subscribers, as compared with Dr Breton's twenty-one votes.[9] These elections were more popularity contests than assessments of medical ability, so the fact that Dr Harrington won the election and held the position for twenty-seven years would suggest that he was an affable and popular figure in the town.

The position of paid medical officer was only a part time appointment, carrying an annual salary of £100, so Dr Harrington maintained his private practice in the town (apparently in partnership with Drs Jamieson and Loftus), while making regular ward rounds and being on call at all times for hospital work. The medical officer was responsible for all patients in the Hospital and performed all operations himself, usually with the assistance of one or more of the honoraries. Dr Harrington frequently referred in his reports to his major operations. For example, in August 1867 he wrote:

> Mr Ford, who has been an inmate of the hospital for some time, suffering from disease of the liver and kidneys, was operated on yesterday for dropsy of the peritoneum. I was kindly assisted by the honorary medical officers of the institution. This day two more operations were performed by me, assisted by the honorary medical officers—one on Wm. Fletcher, for disease of the foot, and the other on John Bogle, who came in this morning. The operation consisted in opening a sinus that existed for two years in the inner aspect of the thigh, close to the groin. Both these operations were performed under the influence of the ether spray with perfect insensibility to pain.[10]

Generally the patients of the Hospital in its early years appear to have been grateful for the attention they received, whatever the outcome, because they were too poor to pay for medical attention and because the public had an understandably pessimistic view of the likely outcome of most medical procedures. Despite this, in June 1867 a patient's father made a complaint against Dr Harrington to the committee. The details were reported in the *Examiner:*

> Edwin Fidler requested the committee to investigate the case of his daughter, alleged to have been admitted into the Hospital with a disease of one eye and discharged incurably blind in both . . . The matron stated that the patient seemed quite blind with one eye and nearly so with the other when admitted. The patient was rather more blind when she left.
>
> Dr Harrington stated that he had treated the patient in a general way to strengthen her constitution, but had not treated her for disease of the eye, which he said he could not cure.
>
> Mr Osburne moved and Mr Cramond seconded: That after investigating the case of Lucinda Fidler, this committee is of opinion that the paid medical officer acted to the best of his judgement in treating the case; at the same time they regret that he did not consult the honorary medical officer in accordance with Rule 13.[11]

The Fidlers took their complaint against Dr Harrington to the courts, with the result that Dr Harrington was exonerated.[12]

There seems to have been some continuing tension between Dr Harrington and the honoraries and the committee frequently reminded the paid medical officer that he should consult with the honoraries on all difficult cases and reminded the honoraries that they should visit the Hospital regularly. This continued throughout Dr Harrington's tenure as paid medical officer. In October 1888 the *Standard* reported on the case of a patient at the Warrnambool Hospital named McFarren, which was "one more illustration of a difference of opinion amongst doctors, and of the patient quietly settling the dispute by betaking himself and his ailment to another world."[13] Mr McFarren had been admitted to the Hospital suffering from hernia, in those days a serious and frequently fatal problem. Dr Harrington called in one of the honoraries, Dr Thomas Scott, who recommended surgery, but "the patient was adverse to the use of the knife" and Dr Harrington also opposed surgery. When the patient died, Dr Scott felt so strongly on the matter that he referred it to the police and an inquest was held. Both doctors were cleared of any mistake, but relations between the two doctors were somewhat strained.

When Dr Harrington retired in 1889 the *Standard* was eloquent in his praise:

> The late paid medical officer is famed far and wide for his almost wonderful surgical skill. The most hopeless cases have never been given up by him, and the knife, when used, was always wielded with the greatest caution. Where a limb would disappear in the twinkling of an eye at the hands of another surgeon, Dr Harrington has always been for giving Dame Nature the first say in the matter, with the result that many a person to this day is stalking about on a sound, though may be contorted limb, . . . owing to the judgement or prescience of the late medical officer.[14]

Following Dr Harrington's retirement the Hospital committee debated the merits of appointing a full time resident medical officer. The *Standard* strongly supported this move in order to enable the Hospital to respond more swiftly when urgent cases were admitted,[15] but the committee felt that it was not yet justified and Dr Linday Miller, a popular local practitioner and member of the Hospital's honorary staff, was appointed to succeed Dr Harrington. Dr Miller's annual salary was set at £100 plus £20 for attendance at the fever ward. It is interesting that this was the same as Dr Harrington had received since the early 1870s, even though the work of the Hospital had greatly increased. In August 1893 Dr Miller applied for his salary to be doubled and the following month the committee agreed to an increase to £130. Dr Miller held the position as paid medical officer until September 1899 when poor health forced his retirement.

Many doctors served the Hospital as honorary medical officers in the years 1860 to 1900, although the number of doctors on the staff fluctuated. In the early 1860s Drs Breton and Singleton shared the position, and in 1870 Dr Jamieson was the sole appointee, while the following year he was joined by Dr Loftus. By the 1880s it had become accepted that the work of the Hospital required at least three honoraries and, at different times, it was assumed that all qualified doctors in the town were de facto honorary medical officers to the Hospital. The role of the honoraries was also unclear. In 1869, for example, Dr Thomas Embling complained that "it was not of much use to appoint honorary medical officers, and to limit them to merely honorary positions, not having even permissive action, but only the power of consultation with the medical officer if he invited them to a conference."[16] In spite of this, the honoraries clearly performed a vital role in the era when the paid medical officer was only part time. The newspapers referred to several cases when the paid medical officer was unavailable to treat emergencies and an honorary doctor was able to respond promptly.[17] It also appears to have been standard practice for an honorary doctor to give anaesthetics for operations at the Hospital, but they were not allowed to usurp the paid medical officer's prerogative of performing surgery.

Doctors who deserve credit for their contribution as honorary medical officers in this period include William Loftus, Thomas Fleetwood, David Jermyn, Lindsay Miller, Thomas Scott, P.J. Macnamara, Frederick Moreton and S.V. Theed. The two most prominent of these in the medical history of the town were Thomas Fleetwood and Thomas Scott. Dr Fleetwood trained in medicine in Ireland and studied in Europe before migrating to Australia in 1874. He came to Warrnambool in 1875, purchased a medical practice and soon after married Susie Rutledge, a member of the prominent pioneering family. He built up a large and successful practice and played a full role in the life of the town, being, among other things, surgeon to the volunteers and a large shareholder in the Ozone Coffee Palace, which he supported as a means of discouraging drunkenness and rioting. In 1890 two of the Fleetwood's children died in a diphtheria epidemic. Dr Fleetwood sold his practice in Warrnambool in 1906 to travel overseas.[18]

Dr Thomas Scott trained in England and Scotland before migrating to Australia in the late 1860s. He established his practice on the corner of Darling and Banyan Streets and, as he became successful, built the private hospital known as "Alveston" on the site. In the late nineteenth and early twentiethth centuries, this was the leading hospital in Warrnambool for those who could afford to pay fees. At the same time, Dr Scott was one of the most active honoraries at Warrnambool Hospital, playing a full role both as consultant and anaesthetist. He retired in the early 1900s and died in 1913.

The period 1860 to 1900 saw major changes in the kinds of treatments used by Warrnambool doctors. At the start of this period "it is probable that a knife or two, a needle or two, and a skein of horsehair in the waistcoat pocket formed their complete surgical outfit, while calomel [protochloride of mercury] was almost a panacea for their medical work."[19] Although the use of anaesthetics had become common, the range of surgical operations was extremely limited as antisepsis was unknown and the mortality from even the most minor operation was very high. Abdominal surgery was believed to be impossible, operations for hernia were considered highly dangerous and a compound fracture was virtually a death sentence. The range of effective drugs was extremely limited and owed more to folk medicine than to science.

By 1900 an understanding of the causes of infection had made a wide range of abdominal surgery possible and formerly hazardous procedures were now considered routine. Although the number of effective drugs had not expanded greatly, many dangerous treatments (such as the use of calomel) had been abandoned, and the new science of bacteriology offered prospects of great progress. One development, which was important in itself as well as foreshadowing further progress, was the introduction of diphtheria anti-toxin in the 1890s. This was invented by Emil Behring in Berlin in 1891 and proved to be highly effective in reducing the mortality from one of the most feared of children's diseases. Warrnambool Hospital gratefully received its first supplies of diphtheria anti-toxin in early 1898, with the committee asking the medical officer to report on its effectiveness, which he soon did in glowing terms.[20]

The progress in surgery was reflected in the reports of the Hospital's medical officer. In 1867 Dr Harrington reported that,

> During the year one of the major operations in surgery was performed (amputation of the leg below the knee). This operation was performed under very unfavourable circumstances, as the friends of the patient removed him from the hospital a few days after the operation was performed, thereby taking away all chance of a favourable result.[21]

By the 1890s, the number of amputations had fallen sharply (as antiseptics greatly lessened the incidence of infection and gangrene following compound fractures) and there was a very low mortality rate for those that were still being performed. Abdominal operations such as appendectomy were being regularly and successfully performed and the repair of hernias, once a life threatening operation, had become a routine procedure.

In spite of the progress in many areas, the medical staff of Warrnambool Hospital were still faced with many illnesses for which they could offer no treatment beyond rest, good food and good nursing. For most common diseases—tuberculosis, typhoid, gastroenteritis, rheumatic fever and, until 1898, diphtheria—doctors had no curative treatments and could only try to relieve the symptoms. The story of the struggle against typhoid in Warrnambool illustrates the problems posed by epidemic infectious disease.

Typhoid appears to have been rare in the early days of Warrnambool; certainly it was not mentioned in the Hospital medical officer's reports or in the local newspapers before the 1870s. However, as the town grew and the pressure increased on water supply and sanitation, the frequency of typhoid epidemics increased. Between 1885 and 1895 scarcely a summer passed without a major typhoid epidemic in the town.

In 1875 Dr James Jamieson published an article in the *Australian Medical Journal* on the treatment of typhoid.[22] It is perhaps an indication of the relative rarity of the disease in Warrnambool at that time that the article is based, not on his own experience of the treatment of that disease, but on the latest ideas in the overseas journals. The significance of the article lies in the nature of the treatments proposed, which represented the forefront of medical science. The recommended treatment can be summarised as being prolonged intensive nursing, with frequent cold baths and application of cold compresses. If the patient became unconscious, Jamieson recommended that "water of 10 °C be poured on the shaven head every half hour as he lies in bed, and the feet are kept wrapped in flannel dipped in hot water. These energetic measures are to be continued as long as the patient breathes, alcoholic stimulants being administered at the same time." Jamieson conceded that these measures did not cut down the fever or significantly reduce the mortality from the disease. For typhoid, as for almost all diseases, medical science in the late nineteenth century could offer no treatment which could cure or even greatly affect the course of the disease. The best doctors could do was to attempt to relieve the symptoms and, with the aid of careful nursing, attempt to help nature complete a cure.

The gradual decline of typhoid from 1893 was not due to a medical breakthrough, but was the result of improved public health measures, particularly the construction of the town's first reticulated water supply. The story of typhoid provides a good example of the strengths and weaknesses of medicine in the late nineteenth century, with great progress in the understanding of the causes of disease, but few major advances in treatments, except for the introduction of antiseptic surgery and, at the very end of the century, diphtheria anti-toxin.

[1] James Jamieson, "On the Parasitic Theory of Disease," *Australian Medical Journal*, August 1876, p.256.
[2] Dr John Day, "On Diphtheria," *Australian Medical Journal*, September 1868, p.266.
[3] Jamieson, "On the Parasitic Theory of Disease," p.256.
[4] Ibid., p.323.
[5] Obituary of James Jamieson in *Medical Journal of Australia*, 9 September 1916, p.218.
[6] John Singleton, *A Narrative of Incidents in the Eventful Life of a Physician*, Melbourne, 1891, p.169.
[7] *Examiner*, 22 January 1864.
[8] *Australian Medical Journal*, March 1872, p.95.
[9] *Examiner*, 14 January 1862.
[10] *Examiner*, 24 August 1867
[11] *Examiner*, 18 June 1867.
[12] *Examiner*, 24 January 1868.
[13] *Standard*, 9 October 1888.
[14] *Standard*, 5 July 1889.
[15] *Standard*, 6 May 1889.
[16] *Examiner*, 18 January 1869.
[17] For example, *Standard*, 6 May 1889.
[18] Information on the career of Thomas Fleetwood from Phillip A. Ritchie, "Thomas Falkner Fleetwood" in Gordon Forth (ed), *The Biographical Dictionary of the Western District of Victoria*, Melbourne, 1998, p.49.
[19] G.T. Howard, "Port Phillip's Early Doctors", in *Medical Journal of Australia*, 17 March 1934, p.366.
[20] *Standard*, 5 February 1898.
[21] *Standarrd*, 19 March 1867.
[22] James Jamieson, "Methods and Results of the Cold-Water Treatment of Typhoid Fever", *Australian Medical Journal*, July 1875.

Chapter 5

NURSES AND THEIR PATIENTS 1860–1900

It is generally recognised today that the recovery of patients in hospitals in the nineteenth century depended far more on the quality of the nursing than the treatments prescribed by the doctors. Despite this we know far more about the doctors than the nurses of this period. This is especially true of Warrnambool Hospital, where very few records of nurses and nursing have survived from before 1900. This is unfortunate, as the second half of the nineteenth century was the period in which hospital nursing underwent a revolution which changed it from an unskilled occupation with no system of training to a profession composed of dedicated and well-trained women occupying a central role in the health system.[1]

It is not possible to assess the extent to which nursing at Warrnambool Hospital in the second half of the nineteenth century followed the same pattern as at other hospitals of that era. It probably did, but we do not know. It is difficult to be absolutely certain even of the names and periods of service of the matrons, and we do not know the names, numbers or any details at all of other nurses before the late 1880s.

In the early days the day to day running of the Hospital and the care of the patients were in the hands of the master and matron and the word "matron" was used interchangeably with "mistress". These positions were normally held by a married couple, who lived at the Hospital and received a single salary. The first master and matron were Mr and Mrs Croll, and they were followed in 1859 by Mr and Mrs Mainwaring. In 1863 the Mainwarings were succeeded by Mr and Mrs Edward Wilson who held their positions for many years. We know little of Mrs Wilson's lengthy term as matron, although she must have run the nursing side of the Hospital with quiet efficiency as she attracted no attention at all in the Hospital's reports and the local press. The Wilsons had fourteen children, but only five survived infancy.

We can only speculate on the nature of patient care during the years in which Mr and Mrs Wilson were responsible. Throughout the 1860s it appears that they personally carried out a high proportion of nursing tasks. The evidence for this is that the total wages paid to other staff was less than £60 and even in an era of very low wages this was probably only enough to employ two or at the most three assistants. We do not know how the various tasks of cooking, cleaning, bed making, admitting and discharging patients, administering medicines, changing bandages, and so on were allocated, but it is certain that Mr and Mrs Wilson must have been both versatile and busy.

The only anecdotes that have come down from the Wilsons' period at the Hospital were told by their daughter, Mrs Charlotte Beattie, shortly before her death in 1953.[2] She believed that her father was "nearly a doctor" as he had done medical training in England, but had not taken out his degree. Many of the Hospital's benevolent patients in those days were old convicts from Van Diemen's Land and Mr Wilson had a large, heavy stick to maintain discipline among them, although he rarely needed to use it. Mrs Beattie recalled that her mother did much of the cooking for the patients and she made beautiful soup as well as jam.

During the 1870s and 1880s Mrs Wilson and her successor, Mrs Maxwell, gradually acquired more assistants as the number of patients grew. These were more probably cooks, cleaners and unskilled servants than what we think of as nurses. One of the few who is named in the records is "Toffie Wilson". In March 1888 the committee noted that he was scarcely fit and decided that he should be given a month's notice and be "replaced by a strong servant".[3] In the same year the first mention is made of a nurse other than the matron, when the committee decided to engage an assistant nurse.[4] It is hard to believe that there were no nurses prior to this date as the Hospital had over thirty inpatients by this time, but the fact remains that there is no evidence of who they were, how many there were, or even whether there were any at all.

Coincidentally, the year 1888 as well as seeing the appointment of an assistant nurse, saw the first recorded problems with the Hospital's matrons. Unfortunately the records are not entirely clear, but the sequence of events seems to have been as follows. Edward and Ellen Wilson held the positions of master and matron with no fuss or bother until Edward Wilson's death in June 1887. John Maxwell of Maryborough Hospital was appointed to succeed Wilson, and, as he was a single man, Mrs Wilson retained her situation as matron. However, this arrangement was unsuccessful. In June 1888 Mr Maxwell made a series of accusations against Mrs Wilson and, after a special meeting at the Town Hall, Mrs Wilson was found guilty by the committee of "insulting conduct, neglect of duty to the sick, not following the instructions of the master, and taking intoxicating drink causing her to become abusive and insulting".[5] She was given six weeks' leave of absence, after which her duties were to cease.

An article in the *Standard* on 2 July 1888 suggests that there were two sides to the story:

> The attempt to dispossess the matron of the Warrnambool Hospital of her position will come as a surprise to the many friends of that lady in this neighbourhood. For the period of a quarter of a century, in company with her late husband, the matron has held her post, without one word of

> complaint as to the manner in which her onerous duties have been carried out. On the death of her husband, the matron was retained in her office. Applications being invited for the position of master, the present gentleman was selected for the position in consequence of his excellent credentials and also for the reason that he was a single man. Since that time the master has become a benedict [got married], though this fact may not be germane to the subject. . . .

In fact, Mrs Wilson's successor as matron was Mrs Maxwell, suggesting that there might well have been a hidden agenda in Mr Maxwell's complaints. It is only fair to record that the committee continued to pay Mrs Wilson for at least six months after her dismissal, in recognition of her long service.

It was during Mrs Maxwell's term as matron that the nurse training school began at the Warrnambool Hospital. This does not seem to have been the result of any formal decision, but rather the response to a growing need for nursing staff. Until the introduction of university training for nurses in the 1980s, most nursing duties at the Hospital were performed by student nurses—this provided a nursing staff at minimal cost, and the trainees gained a valuable qualification while receiving free board and some pay.

The first reference to nurse training came in September 1895 when the master suggested that "a probationer be appointed for 1–2 years to be trained as a nurse."[6] The following month the secretary reported that Marie Stewart had been engaged as a probationary nurse for two years with an allowance for a uniform in the first year and pay of £8 for the second year. We know nothing of the training Miss Stewart received, but it was certainly more practical than theoretical and would have involved a large amount of hard physical work and very long hours. She completed her training successfully in October 1897 and was retained on the staff at the increased annual salary of £18, with the promise of a permanent position when a vacancy occurred on the nursing staff.

The increased number of nurses and the beginning of nurse training at the Hospital prompted a member of the committee, Mr Bryant, to suggest that better provision should be made for the accommodation of the nursing staff. However, although the committee voted to treat this as a matter of urgency, nothing seems to have come of it in the short term.[7]

In January 1862 the first annual report of Warrnambool Hospital after the opening of the new building in Ryot Street, in May 1861, noted that the Hospital had admitted sixty-five inpatients during the year and the average number of inpatients in the Hospital was fourteen. There were eighteen "out-door patients" on the Hospital's books, as well as thirteen families with thirty-two children who received outdoor relief in the form of food or money from the Benevolent Society. The Hospital also "forwarded 13 patients to Melbourne, who, in most instances, have returned cured," though it is not clear where in Melbourne they were sent. Dr Breton, the paid medical officer, reported that he had treated seventy-three patients during the year of whom forty-nine had been cured, sixty-one discharged, five died and eight remained in hospital.

By the end of the century the Hospital was treating as many patients in a month as it had in a year in the early 1860s. In early February 1900 the medical officer reported that there were seventy patients in the Hospital, with twenty-one admitted, seventeen discharged and five deaths in the previous month.[8] In neither 1862 nor 1900 was there a breakdown of the numbers of benevolent patients and hospital patients, but it is clear that the emphasis was increasingly on caring for the sick rather than providing a refuge for the aged poor. Nonetheless it is important to remember that in the years before 1900, the Hospital accepted only poor people as patients. With the exceptions only of emergency cases and, from the mid-1880s, a very small number of paying patients, all the Hospital's patients had to demonstrate their inability to pay for medical treatment.

Apart from the matrons, Marie Stewart is the only nurse we know the name of before 1900. However, the local press and the committee minutes contain many anecdotes of patients, enabling us to gain some picture of the people the Hospital was built to serve. We have accounts of the victims of accidents, of people suffering from dropsy, phthisis, colonial fever, housemaid's knee, and other ailments not spoken of these days, as well as asthma, cancer, hepatitis and other more familiar ailments.

The pattern of accidents in the late nineteenth century was very different from today. Most accidents reported in the local press involved horses, with farm accidents being the next biggest group. Chaff-cutting machines were involved in many accidents, as in this report:

> An inquest was held by Dr Harrington, District Coroner, on the body of Peter M'Farlane Breingen, who died at Tooram on the previous day.
>
> . . . J. Fulton, a stock rider, in the employ of Mr Orlebar, said that the deceased, who had worked on the same farm for three years, was a young man about sixteen years of age; that he was on the shaft of the chaff cutter, and got his leg jammed between the frame and the shaft. . . .
>
> John Sharp, also employed on the Tooram farm, deposed that the boy had slammed the whip when driving two horses in the chaff cutting machine; one of them made a jump, which threw the deceased off the pole. He (the witness) at once removed the lad to his mother's house and sent for Dr Mackenzie.
>
> Dr Boyd informed the jury that he and Dr Mackenzie went out to Tooram, and found the deceased lying on a stretcher in his mother's house. He was suffering from a lacerated wound of the right leg and thigh, about six inches in length. There was a compound dislocation of the knee joint. The haemorrhage was considerable, and the boy was greatly prostrated. He and Dr Mackenzie agreed that amputation was necessary, as the only means of saving life. After he had administered chloroform, the thigh was amputated by Dr Mackenzie about the middle. Both of them paid every attention to their patient and used every remedy, but the shock and loss of blood were too great. The boy was very weak, but quite sensible, before the operation.[9]

This story illustrates the dangers of farm work at the time, the problem of obtaining medical help following an accident, the difficulty of getting patients to hospital and the conditions in which the Hospital's honorary doctors were sometimes forced to operate.

An area in which there was great progress in surgery in the last decades of the nineteenth century was the treatment of compound fractures. Prior to the introduction of Lister's antiseptic methods a compound fracture was normally followed by amputation and frequently death, but by the 1880s, most patients recovered completely. In January 1888 the *Standard* reported on another farm accident:

> An exceedingly painful accident happened to a young man named Harry Duner, a Swede, employed by Mr W. Anderson, M.L.A. at Rosemount. A threshing machine was at work on the farm, and Duner was engaged at work on the adjacent stack of hay. When the whistle blew to call the men to dinner he commenced to come down, when two of the sheaves slipped from under him, and he fell into the machine, which was fortunately being slackened off at the time, and was stopped with all possible haste. Duner was then rescued from his very dangerous position and it was found that he had sustained severe injuries. He was at once conveyed to the Hospital where he was examined by Dr Harrington, who found that the injured man had sustained a compound fracture of the left leg, and the foot was also severely crushed. The fractured leg was set, and everything possible was done to alleviate the patient's sufferings, and he is now progressing as favourably as possible.[10]

Harry Duner was in hospital for many months (leading to a dispute between the Hospital and Mr Anderson over the expenses incurred in his treatment) but he eventually made a good recovery, with full use of his leg.

For many years the local papers printed reports of all deaths in the Hospital and these reports give an interesting picture of the patients and the diseases they suffered from. This random selection indicates the high proportion of single men in the community, the low life expectancy of the period, and the prevalence of alcoholism:

> On Friday last, a patient who has been some time in the hospital, and who was a labouring man well known in the town as Edward Pruin (or Terrible Teddy) died from dropsy. He was a native of Middlesex, England, and was about 44 years of age, and was generally believed to be unmarried.[11]
>
> On Saturday last, an old man named John Pickering, better known as "Old Jock" or "Scotch Jock" died in the hospital. He was only admitted on Christmas Day. Enlargement of the heart was the cause of death. The deceased was a single man, 60 years of age, a native of Liddesdale, Scotland, religious profession, Presbyterian, and had been 40 years in the colony.[12]
>
> A death occurred on the 8th instant in the Warrnambool Hospital. The deceased's name was William Russell, aged 64, from Woodford Forest. He had been a resident in the colony for thirty-nine years, and died from paralysis.[13]

Another death has occurred in the hospital. The following particulars will afford some information to deceased's friends:- James Shields, 41, single, labourer, native of Galway, Ireland, Roman Catholic, seven years in the colony, had been working for Mr Gibson, Tower Hill. Admitted 15th December 1866, died 25th January 1867, cause of death, broken down constitution.[14]

Two patients died in the hospital on Saturday last. The following are the particulars:- William Thomas, 33, single, labourer, residence Warrnambool, native of Wales, religion, Church of England, nine years in the colony, admitted 2nd April 1867, died 8th June, cause of death: water on the chest. Lawrence Murphy, 60, married, ship's carpenter, residence Yallock, native place Yorkshire, England, religion Church of England, 42 years in the colony, admitted 22nd May, died 8th June, cause of death: enlargement of the liver.[15]

A death is reported as having occurred in the hospital on the 6th inst. The deceased was Richard Burrows, who was brought down from Mortlake on the evening of the 4th. He had been suffering from "strangulated hernia" since Christmas, when his complaint was brought on by immoderate fits of laughter. His medical attendants had failed to reduce the hernia, but this was done by Dr Harrington in a few minutes. Mortification, however, set in, and the case terminated fatally. He was forty-seven years of age, a native of Bedfordshire, and by trade a gardener. He was a married man and had been only five months in the colony.[16]

A man named Patrick O'Shea died in the Warrnambool Hospital on Sunday morning. The deceased was admitted to the institution on the 6th instant, suffering from *delirium tremens* and an ulcerated leg. He was well attended by Dr Harrington, but the constitution of the poor fellow had been so undermined by hard drinking, that medical skill proved of no avail, and the sufferer gradually sank and died at the early age of 29. He had been employed for some time as a gardener by Mr A. Tobin, at Yalloak Station, and was formerly an industrious hard-working man.[17]

Another group of patients whose stories are preserved are those who were problems for the Hospital management. Most of these seem to have come from among the benevolent patients, the aged poor who made up probably half the patients in the period 1861 to 1900. The greatest problem among the benevolent patients was drunkenness. In 1875, for example, six patients were discharged for drunkenness during the year and, although the figures are not given for every year, it seems that this was fairly typical.

However, the committee of management was remarkably tolerant of the behaviour of many of its patients and went to great lengths to ensure that they were well cared for. The story of Patrick Dunne illustrates this. On 5 January 1884 he returned to the Hospital after going on the spree with friends over Christmas, but was refused admittance for breaking the rules and, "having nowhere to go, gave himself up to the police, who charged him with vagrancy".[18] The committee relented and readmitted Mr Dunne, but in August 1885 the minutes noted: "Patient P. Dunne not to be admitted again on account of his gross misconduct." For the next four months members of the committee tried very hard to find alternative accommodation for him and, in January 1886 they succeeded in obtaining him a place in the Benevolent Asylum in Melbourne. Unfortunately, Patrick Dunne's behaviour proved as unacceptable in Melbourne as it had in Warrnambool with the result that he was returned to Warrnambool within two months. Rather than readmit him, the committee decided to give him five shillings a week to enable him to live outside the Hospital. We hear no more of Patrick Dunne and can only hope that he settled down to a life of sobriety.

There are few stories in the surviving records of the patients who were treated successfully and discharged—although even in the nineteenth century most patients survived a stay in hospital. One success story was that of

> Mrs Court, who was admitted into hospital on 13th of May, for a badly treated fracture of both bones of the leg, which took place six months before up country. The leg presented a most formidable appearance, it was about twice its natural size, and she could not put it to the ground. At one time amputation was thought of, but by rest and good constitutional treatment, in six weeks she was able to leave the Institution, and walk home with the aid of a stick, to her great delight. She expressed herself in the highest terms of gratitude for the benefit derived, considering the short time she was in the Hospital, viz., six weeks.[19]

[1] The revolution in nursing between 1850 and 1900 is described in Brian Abel-Smith, *A History of the Nursing Profession*, London, 1960, chs1–3; and Elizabeth Burchill, *Australian Nurses Since Nightingale, 1860–1990*, Melbourne, 1992, chs1–2.
[2] *Standard*, 12 October 1953.
[3] Committee of Management Minutes, March 1888.
[4] Committee of Management Minutes, November 1888.
[5] Committee of Management Minutes, June and July 1888.
[6] Committee of Management Minutes, September 1895.
[7] Committee of Management Minutes, March 1898.
[8] *Standard*, 11 February 1900.
[9] *Examiner*, 22 November 1867.
[10] *Standard*, 27 January 1888.
[11] *Examiner*, 26 January 1866.
[12] *Examiner*, 1 January 1867.
[13] *Examiner*, 11 October 1867.
[14] *Examiner*, 1 February 1867.
[15] *Examiner*, 11 June 1867.
[16] *Examiner*, 12 January 1869.
[17] *Standard*, 11 January 1870.
[18] *Standard*, 5 January 1884.
[19] *Examiner*, 23 July 1867.

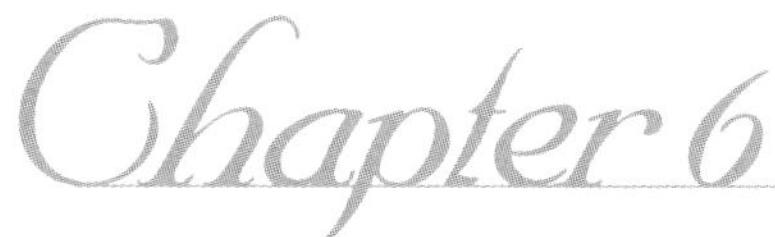

THE HOSPITAL REMADE: COMMITTEE, BUILDING AND FINANCES, 1860–1900

The period 1900 to 1939 was an era of war, depression and stagnation in many areas of Australian society. By contrast, for the Warrnambool Hospital this period saw a fundamental realignment, which turned it from a charity hospital whose main purpose was to care for the aged poor into a modern hospital catering for the whole community. Two major building projects totally changed its physical appearance and provided for the first time maternity and children's wards, a modern operating theatre, x-ray facilities and a pathology laboratory. The role of government in hospital funding grew rapidly, being supplemented by new local initiatives, in particular the development of the Hospital auxiliaries. The driving force behind these developments was Marcus Saltau, the greatest figure in the Hospital's history, who served as president in 1904–05 and from 1912 to 1941.

Marcus Saltau was born in Warrnambool in 1869 and, after leaving school at the age of fifteen, he began work in his father's thriving produce and shipping business. He ran the business very successfully for many years. Marcus Saltau was a leader of many community endeavours, being inaugural chairman of the Warrnambool Chamber of Commerce, playing a leading role in the foundation of the Warrnambool Woollen Mill and being largely responsible for the decision by Nestlé to build its milk condensery at Dennington. He was an active member of the congregation of St John's Presbyterian Church.

Ironically, the first mention of Marcus Saltau in the records of the Warrnambool Hospital came in February 1896 when the committee of management minutes noted that Mr Marcus Saltau's daughter had been treated as an inpatient and the account of £5 for her treatment had been ignored. Six months later the account was still unpaid and was placed in the hands of a solicitor, with what result we do not know.[1] This incident cannot have led to any long term bad feeling as Marcus Saltau joined the Hospital committee in 1899 and from the start was one of the committee's most active and enthusiastic members, serving as president in 1904 and 1905. Shortly after retiring as president, he moved that the committee consider building a maternity ward, a children's ward, and a pharmacy. These seemingly obvious constituents of an efficient hospital aroused the

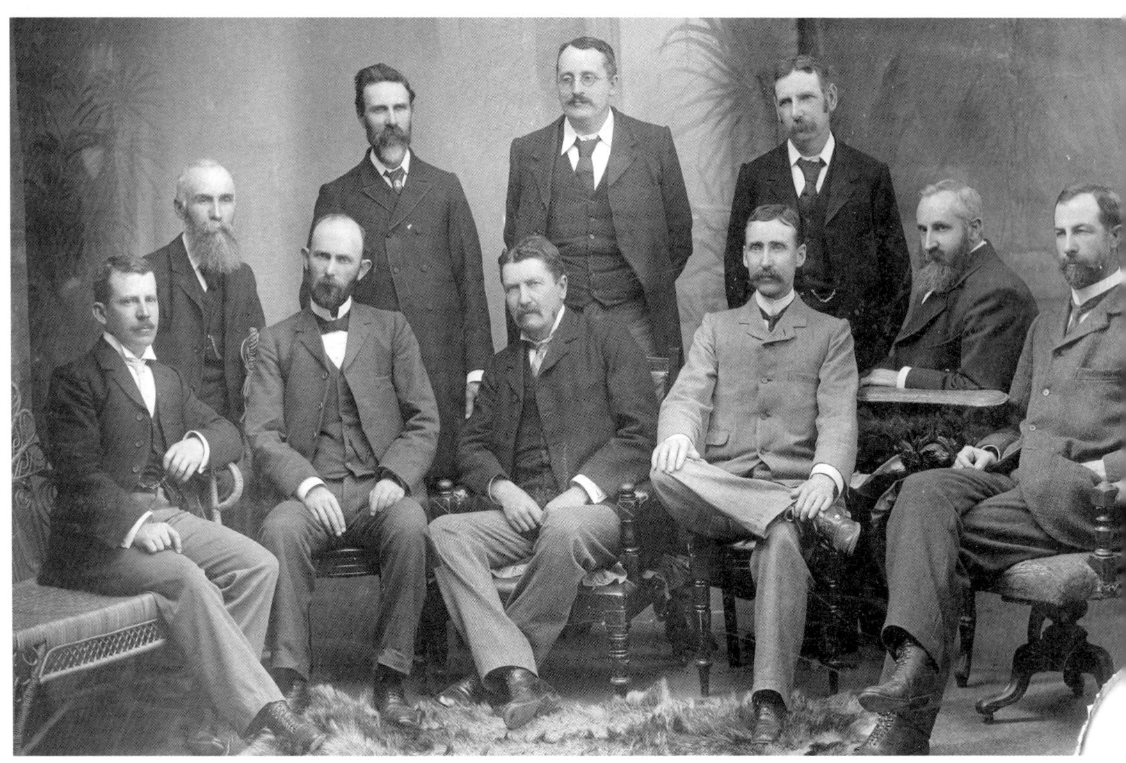

Board of management, 1908

opposition of many members of the committee (for reasons which will be discussed later), and it took Marcus Saltau many years of effort before he succeeded in gaining support for these developments.

In 1912 Marcus Saltau was re-elected to the presidency, and held the position for the next twenty-nine years. This lengthy term of office saw the Hospital surmount the challenges of the First World War and the Depression, and, with the completion of two major building projects and a total change in admission policies and financial structure, become a modern regional hospital. Although Mr Saltau resided primarily in Melbourne following his election to parliament in 1925, he missed very few committee meetings and was automatically re-elected president every year until ill-health forced him to retire in 1941, four years before his death. Marcus Saltau held such a pre-eminent place in the life of Warrnambool and the work of the Hospital that it is difficult to find an objective assessment of his personality. Airlie Worrall, the author of the entry on Marcus Saltau in the *Australian Dictionary of Biography*, noted that "The *Warrnambool Standard* admired his geniality and his tact in handling men and affairs, but to his fellow hospital committee-men he seems to have appeared autocratic and overbearing."[2] Whatever the assessment of his personality, the reality of his enormous contribution cannot be exaggerated and, if he appeared to some to be "autocratic and overbearing", then this was a small price to pay for the progress he brought about through his energy and enthusiasm.

The personality of Marcus Saltau overshadowed the working of the committee of management throughout the period 1900 to 1939, and few other personalities stand out. The makeup of the committee remained essentially as it had been in the late nineteenth century, with almost all committee members coming from Warrnambool's business and professional elite. The committee was still exclusively male and membership was seen as one of the community service obligations which then were accepted as part of membership of the town's elite. Among the long-serving members of the Hospital committee in this period were James Dickson, of Cramond and Dickson's, William Ardlie, solicitor, H.H. Smith, businessman and long-serving municipal councillor, J.D.E. Walter, builder and developer, J.McD. Taylor, solicitor, and E.A. Wright, car dealer.

The reshaping of the Warrnambool Hospital under the leadership of Marcus Saltau was not a straightforward process. Particularly in the years before the First World War, there was strong opposition to change. The critical issue over which the reformers and the conservatives fought was the proposal to establish a maternity ward. In this era almost all babies were born at home, normally with the attendance only of a midwife, most of whom were untrained. The Hospital normally only saw the midwives' failures, frequently too late to alter the outcome. The proposal that the Hospital make some provision for births was first made in January 1901, when four doctors suggested that one or two beds be made available for "deserving midwifery cases". However, a motion to establish a "lying-in ward" was defeated by ten votes to four. Four years later, Marcus Saltau raised the issue again, combining it with a proposal to erect a children's ward and a dispensary and this time the issue was fully debated at a special meeting in December 1905. The arguments in favour of the proposal were voiced by Marcus Saltau, who told the meeting that he could point out a dozen cases "of the most harrowing character" to show the need for a maternity ward, and he was supported by Mr Hickford who stated that there had been a need for a maternity ward for years.

Although C.E. Sayers has stated that the opposition to accepting midwifery cases was based on the belief that this would tend to "condone or induce community immorality", he did not give his source for this statement and the present author has been unable to substantiate it.[3] The arguments presented at the special meeting against the proposal were that it would be too expensive and was not needed. William Ardlie summarised these when he said: "There is no point in establishing a maternity ward and then finding we have no funds. Married women have managed all right in this district without a maternity ward." He concluded that he did not want to appear less humane than his friends, but it was only since the maternity ward was mentioned that these cases of hardship arose.[4] On this occasion, the committee actually affirmed the principle of establishing a maternity ward, but a meeting of subscribers called in March 1906 rejected the proposal and it was not raised again for many years,

The years 1900 to 1914 were among the most turbulent in the history of the Hospital, with many controversies and rapid turnover of senior staff. The situation in this period is epitomised by the turmoil in the once stable position of master. The long-serving master and matron partnership of Mr and Mrs Maxwell served until Mr Maxwell's ill health forced their retirement in 1901. Mr J. Stewart was appointed in his place, but within weeks was reported as suffering from "fits" (with a strong innuendo they were produced by alcohol), and he was sacked. Several more short term appointments followed, during which the title steward was substituted for master, and, from 1908 the position was combined with that of hospital dispenser. The first holder of this combined position was George Colquhoun, who had not held the post for long when an examination of the books showed "irregularities"—money received from patients had not been deposited in the bank and several of the staff had not been paid their salaries, while the salary cheques of others had been dishonoured by the bank. Colquhoun pleaded guilty to larceny and his position was taken by a Mr Gall. In 1910, for the first time, the positions of secretary and steward were combined, with Mr Gall receiving the position, although he did not stay long, resigning in May 1910.

The turnover of matrons and senior nursing staff was similarly rapid and the committee of management minutes for these years give the impression that the committee was too busily engaged sorting out crises to consider issues of long term planning. The situation showed clear signs of improving after Marcus Saltau began his long term presidency in 1912, but any major projects had to be put aside in 1914 following the outbreak of the First World War.

The First World War did not have nearly as great an impact on the everyday operation of the Warrnambool Hospital as the Second World War. Beyond putting any major building projects on hold, the major problems were staff shortages, particularly of doctors, as many of the honorary staff volunteered for service and it became very difficult to obtain resident medical officers. Although many nurses volunteered for service overseas, including the matron, Miss Reeves, there was never a serious shortage of nurses as many more young women saw nursing as the best way to serve in wartime.

Immediately following the War, the Hospital was confronted with the most serious epidemic in its history, in the form of the Spanish influenza pandemic, which caused more deaths around the world than the First World War. The response of the Hospital's medical and nursing staff will be discussed in greater detail in the following chapters, but the impact of the influenza epidemic certainly slowed the implementation of any major projects.

As a result of this succession of obstacles and delays, by the early 1920s the Warrnambool Hospital was becoming seriously inadequate and out of date. This was recognised in the 1919 Annual Report which pointed out

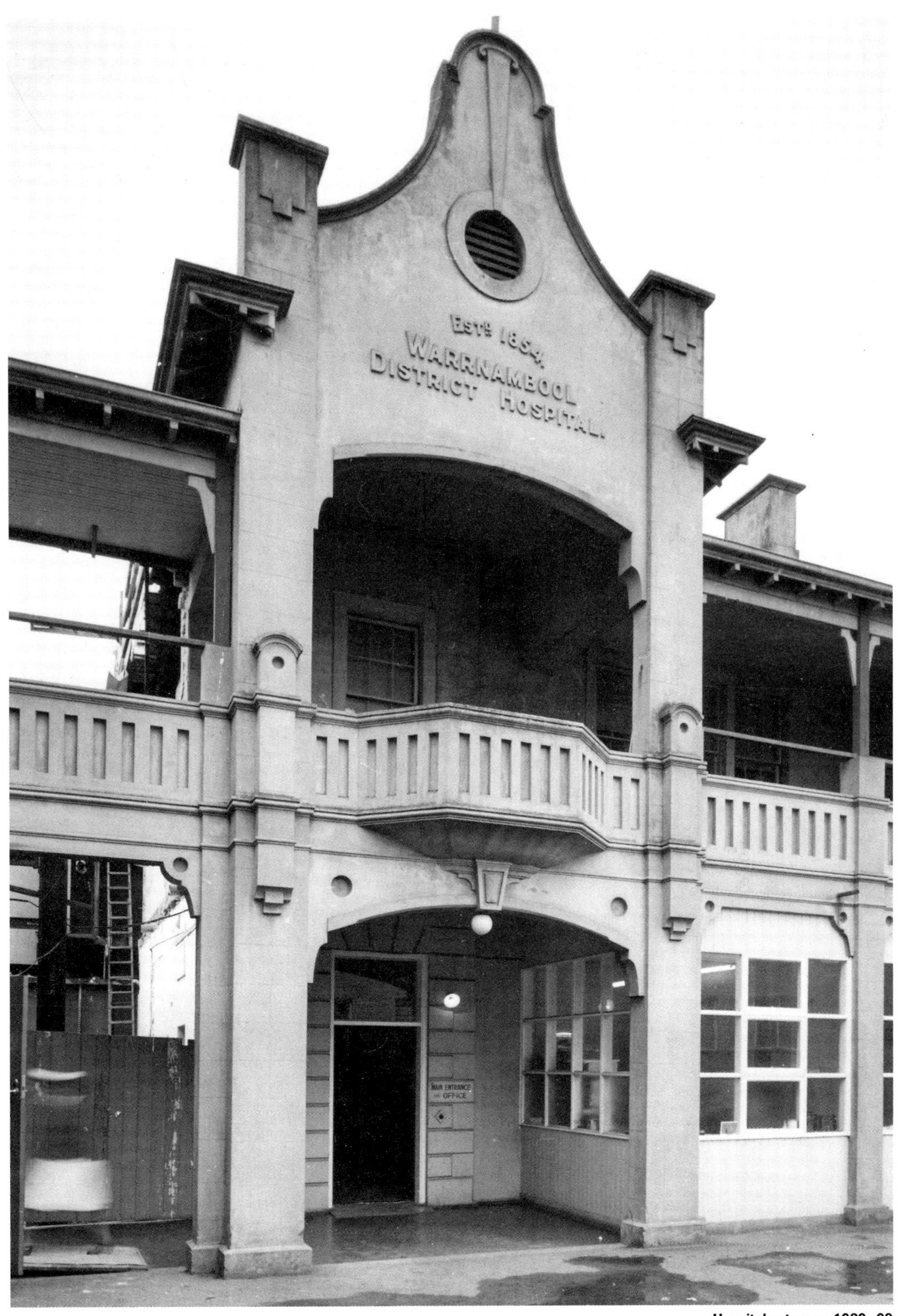

Hospital entrance, 1929–63

that a large amount of money was required for urgent renovations and repairs and to provide a new operating theatre, an x-ray department, a major updating of the laundry, steam service to the wards and "for a general remodelling of the Hospital". The report expressed the belief that the Warrnambool Hospital should be the centre for the provision of health care services to the region, but in its current state this was impossible and many patients had to be sent to Melbourne because of the lack of modern equipment.

The 1919 Annual Report also formally announced that the Hospital would no longer cater for benevolent patients. Whereas in the early years of its history, the role of asylum for the aged poor was paramount, by the later years of the nineteenth century the proportion of benevolent patients had fallen sharply and fewer were admitted. In 1919 the committee announced that only five benevolent patients remained and it recommended that "Separate provision should be made, quite apart from the Hospital, for these old folk." No more patients were admitted simply on the grounds of being old and poor and by 1925 the Hospital had become purely medical and surgical.

The physical rebuilding which took place under Marcus Saltau's leadership occurred in two phases, one ending in 1928 and the next in 1938, with the Depression intervening. The first phase began in 1920, when the Hospital received a bequest of £1000 from the estate of George Rolfe, "the squire of Lyndoch", and a further £1000 from his step-daughters, Anne and Florence Lake. Supplementing this with an energetic fundraising campaign, the Hospital raised the money for the George Rolfe operating theatre and x-ray unit, a children's ward, a new laundry, laboratories and, finally, a maternity ward. Marcus Saltau himself donated £500 toward the building of the maternity ward, which was named the Jean Buick Saltau ward in memory of his wife. The final stage of this phase of rebuilding was completed in 1928 and, at the opening ceremony, the Inspector of Charities, Mr R.J. Love, said, "They had now in Warrnambool an institution that could be favourably compared with anything of its kind anywhere in structure, equipment and general efficient service".[5]

In spite of the praise the Hospital committee received for the major projects of the 1920s, Marcus Saltau argued strongly that more needed to be done to make the Warrnambool Hospital a truly modern base hospital for the region. The greatest need was to make some provision for what were described at the time as "intermediate" patients. As the *Standard* pointed out in an editorial in 1935, the existing hospital system did not cater at all for "the great middle section of the community", as the public hospitals were only for the poor, while the cost of private hospitals made them inaccessible to all but the very well off.[6] The answer appeared to lie in the provision of "intermediate" wards at public hospitals, in which the patient would pay both hospital and medical fees, but at a lesser rate than in private hospitals.

The response of the Warrnambool Hospital committee was the construction of Marcus Saltau House, to provide for both private and intermediate patients as well as for greatly expanded maternity services, as the use of the first maternity ward had been so great. The new construction also involved new kitchens, built on the site of the old male ward, and the construction of a new male ward. Ernie Harris was the contractor for Marcus Saltau house, which, at the time, reflected the latest thinking in hospital design. This phase of the Hospital's redevelopment also included a new nurses' home, which was designed by W.J.T. Walter, a young Warrnambool architect, and was completed before the outbreak of war in 1939.

In July 1939, just weeks before the beginning of the Second World War, J.L. Plummer, the secretary of the Warrnambool Base Hospital (as it was known by then) gave an address to the Warrnambool Apex Club in which he outlined the progress of the Hospital. After noting that the number of patients treated annually had trebled in the previous decade, Mr Plummer said,

> The Base Hospital was now caring for 115 in-patients, to all of whom, regardless of creed, colour or financial standing, unexcelled treatment was available. Every Warrnambool doctor was an honorary medical officer, and, in addition to 65 nurses, the staff included a qualified chemist and an experienced dietician. Approximately 300 babies were ushered into the world annually at the Hospital.
>
> Modern improvements include a self-contained telephone network, a paging system and electrically heated trolleys which ensure meals reaching patients at the same heat as they leave the kitchen.
>
> Although £52,000 had been spent on additions and improvements during the past two years, the finances of the Warrnambool Hospital were in an unusually healthy condition as compared to most Victorian public hospitals.[7]

[1] Committee of Management Minutes, February and October 1896.

[2] Airlie Worrall, "Marcus Saltau", *Australian Dictionary of Biography*, 11, p.513.

[3] Sayers and Yule, *By These We Flourish*, p.164. Peter Yule would like to note that the research and writing of the history of the Hospital given in chapter 17 of *By These We Flourish* was solely the work of the late C.E. Sayers.

[4] Committee of Management Minutes, 28 December 1905.

[5] *Standard*, 30 November 1928.

[6] *Standard*, 22 February 1935.

[7] *Standard*, 9 June 1939.

Chapter 7

COMMUNITY INVOLVEMENT: JAM, EGGS AND WOOD

Before 1900 a large proportion of the work of the Warrnambool Hospital was concerned with the care of old people who were in the Hospital because they were poor rather than because they were sick. The care of the aged poor was considerably less expensive than the care of the seriously ill and this fact became very important as the Hospital became a purely medical institution. A consequence was that the period 1900 to 1914 was an era of stagnation at the Warrnambool Hospital. Although many ideas were advanced for major projects and suggestions made for important innovations, few reached fruition, primarily because of shortage of funds. The financial structure of the Hospital had arisen in the benevolent asylum days and was not suited to the changing function of the institution. Before the committee of management could undertake modernisation, it had to establish a financial base which could sustain the construction of new buildings, the purchase and maintenance of modern equipment and the care and treatment of seriously ill patients.

In the benevolent asylum era the Hospital had relied on two main sources of finance, an annual government grant and subscriptions from the better-off citizens of the town and district. When the Hospital was faced with a major financial outlay, the community could be relied on to support a special effort, but there was no continuing means of maintaining community involvement and there were long periods of public apathy.

As the committee began modernising, it began to explore alternative sources of finance. The most obvious of these was the Government, and the period 1900 to 1939 did see a large increase in the level of government funding of all hospitals.

The increase in government funding was part of a greater commitment of government to the provision of health care in the state and was not dependent on local initiative, but the Warrnambool Hospital committee supplemented this with a large increase in the amount of its income which was raised locally, and this came from a far higher and more consistent level of community involvement.

The committee was aware from the early 1900s that it must make a greater effort to attract support from the town and the district, but there were several false starts before this was achieved. In the late nineteenth century it was normal practice for hospitals to employ "collectors" to raise funds on a commission basis, but this system does not appear to have been adopted in Warrnambool. There was a proposal to employ a collector in 1860, but it does not appear to have proceeded, and for the rest of the century most local fundraising was carried out by committee members with the support of the local press. It was natural, therefore, that when the committee began to look for new ways of raising money that it should see the appointment of a collector as the logical first step. The committee called for applications for a collector to receive a base salary of £15 plus a commission of twenty per cent of monies collected and, in November 1906, Stanley Williams was appointed. Very high hopes were held of this appointment, with one committee man suggesting that the collector would raise subscriptions from the existing level of about £300 to £1300.[1] However, the results of this appointment were extremely disappointing. Mr Williams had raised only £20 before his services were dispensed with in June 1907, and, while his successor, Mr Fulton, did a little better, he still raised only £147 in his first full year. Following Mr Fulton's resignation, George Edwards was appointed collector in May 1910, but he was no more successful than his predecessor and was given notice in July 1911. The committee then abandoned the attempt to raise money through paid collectors and returned to the system of voluntary fundraising by committee members with the aid of honorary collectors in country districts.[2]

The First World War saw great pressure on the finances as the government grant was reduced and local fundraising was devoted primarily to patriotic causes. The committee only succeeded in nursing the Hospital through the crisis by means of strict economy on expenditure, increased contributions from patients, some well-timed bequests and some novel fundraising methods, such as the voluntary donation of one penny a week by every employee of the Warrnambool Woollen Mill.

With the end of the War the Hospital was faced with the problems of making up for years of skimping on expenditure during the War, as well as making provision for the extensive modernisation scheme envisaged by Marcus Saltau. The committee relied firstly on large scale public appeals to raise money for capital expenditure and secondly on a great increase in donations of goods and services to reduce the pressure on maintenance expenditure.

The Warrnambool Base Hospital held three major building appeals in the inter-war years. These were highly organised, well supported by the *Standard* and all reached their fairly ambitious targets. The first appeal was launched in 1920 and the first function, a market day, raised the extraordinary total of £5298. The target of the appeal was set at £10,000, but it finally raised closer to £20,000. The second appeal beginning in 1929 was not as successful, due to the onset of the Depression, but it still succeeded in raising enough money to pay the outstanding debts on the major building projects of the 1920s. The final appeal before the Second World War was launched to pay the local contribution toward the cost of Marcus Saltau House and the other major capital works of the late 1930s. It had the relatively modest target of £5000, which was easily reached.

More interesting than the large scale appeals (important as they were), was the great rise in the level of donations of goods and services, primarily through the newly formed hospital auxiliaries, and the increased level of community participation in the Hospital this encouraged. The pioneer of these new forms of community involvement was the egg appeal which began in a small way in 1910, and grew rapidly in the post-war years. By the mid-1920s the Hospital was receiving its entire requirements of eggs in the egg appeal, with literally thousands of dozens being donated. The egg appeal was particularly strongly promoted in the schools of Warrnambool and district, with many tiny rural schools donating generously. In 1926, for example, the Hospital acknowledged donations of forty-eight dozen by Cooramook State School, thirty dozen by Mepunga East, twenty-four dozen by Woolsthorpe, twenty-three dozen by Hopkins Point, twenty-two dozen by Winslow, twenty-one dozen by Mailor's Flat and eighteen dozen by Dennington, among many others.[3] At the conclusion of the appeal, the *Standard* noted that the eggs were "put in the preserving tanks for the use of the institution until the egg season next year".[4]

It is unclear where the idea for hospital auxiliaries started, but they began in many hospitals around Australia in the years after the First World War. It seems likely that the feeling of community participation engendered by the Red Cross and similar organisations during the war was redirected in peacetime to supporting local hospitals.[5]

The exact chronology of the formation of the Warrnambool Hospital auxiliaries is not entirely clear. A brief history of the Warrnambool Base Hospital Senior Ladies Auxiliary compiled by Mrs N. Moore states that that auxiliary originated with the Red Cross Hospital Auxiliary in 1923,[6] while the Hospital's annual report for 1924–25 states that, "The Red Cross Auxiliary was formed and was doing excellent work," suggesting a later origin. However, other evidence suggests an earlier date, with the numbering of the auxiliaries' annual meetings suggesting that they began in 1921—the 1928 meeting being labelled as the seventh annual meeting and so on.[7]

The Warrnambool Hospital auxiliaries developed from the wartime work of the Red Cross, when the members decided to extend their charitable work to include the Hospital. Before long the Hospital became the main focus for their work, most of which consisted of providing goods and services for the Hospital rather than cash donations. The report of the auxiliary's annual meeting of 1928 gives a good picture of the work carried out in this era:

> Mrs Jackman read the annual report, which was as follows:-
>
> During the year the ladies have maintained the keen interest in the Auxiliary and have attended to the work in a most enthusiastic manner. The sewing bees were well attended, and during the year the following

articles were provided: 62 hucka towels, 15 surgeons' gowns, 3 glove sasha, 23 quilts, 36 towels, 8 binders, 24 tea towels, 166 sheets, 9 tray cloths, a number of belts and covers . . . As in past years the ladies of the Auxiliary launched the annual jam appeal in February last and the response was most satisfactory—some hundreds of jars of jam and honey being placed in the Hospital pantry . . . Reports were received from Grassmere, Allansford, Dennington, Nullawarre, and Wangoom, all of which showed that good work had been done and that the country centres had supplied the Hospital with a quantity of goods, crockery and supplies of various kinds.

In the early days, the main role of the auxiliaries was to make bedspreads, gowns, napkins and sheets and for many years they provided a high proportion of the Hospital's needs. The auxiliaries did carry out some fundraising, mainly through street stalls, in order to purchase materials to make up for the Hospital, but from the late 1930s the Hospital began to purchase the materials for the auxiliaries to make up.

A very large number of women from Warrnambool and district contributed to the work of the auxiliaries in the inter-war years. Among the most prominent leaders of the auxiliaries at this time were Mrs J.D.E. Walter, Mrs H.J. Worland, Mrs W.L. Marfell, Miss Doherty, Miss McCullough and Mrs Abbey. The work of the auxiliaries was important not just for the very substantial contribution of goods and services they made, but for the increased feeling of community involvement in the Hospital they encouraged. As people worked for the Hospital they came increasingly to think of it as "their" hospital. Marcus Saltau was very aware of this and he worked hard to encourage the development of the concept of a "community hospital" rather than the previous image of a charity hospital.[8]

The increasing level of community involvement with the Hospital was shown in many ways during the 1920s and 1930s. A good example of this was the provision of wood supplies to the Hospital during the Depression years in the early 1930s. The *Standard* told the story:

The proposal to organise "wood days" for the Warrnambool and District Base Hospital and thus relieve the institution of the necessity of paying out something like £220 a year for the purchase of the commodity has been taken up enthusiastically by a number of city and country residents. The proposal emanated from the local group of Toc H, and following a meeting . . . when Councillor P.R. Le Couteur generously offered to allow sufficient wood to be cut on his property at Boggy Creek for the coming year, another meeting was held at the Market Buildings on Wednesday afternoon which was attended by many residents from different centres surrounding Warrnambool as well as members of Toc H and the Hospital Committee . . .

Mr Fletcher Jones was chosen as organising secretary . . . and the following gentlemen were appointed a committee: Messrs Jas. Burleigh, F. Hesketh, P.R. Le Couteur, R. Milne, D. Hogan, R. Batten and C. Gordon.

Many other landowners offered access to their properties to cut wood, and a large number of volunteers from around the district formed working bees

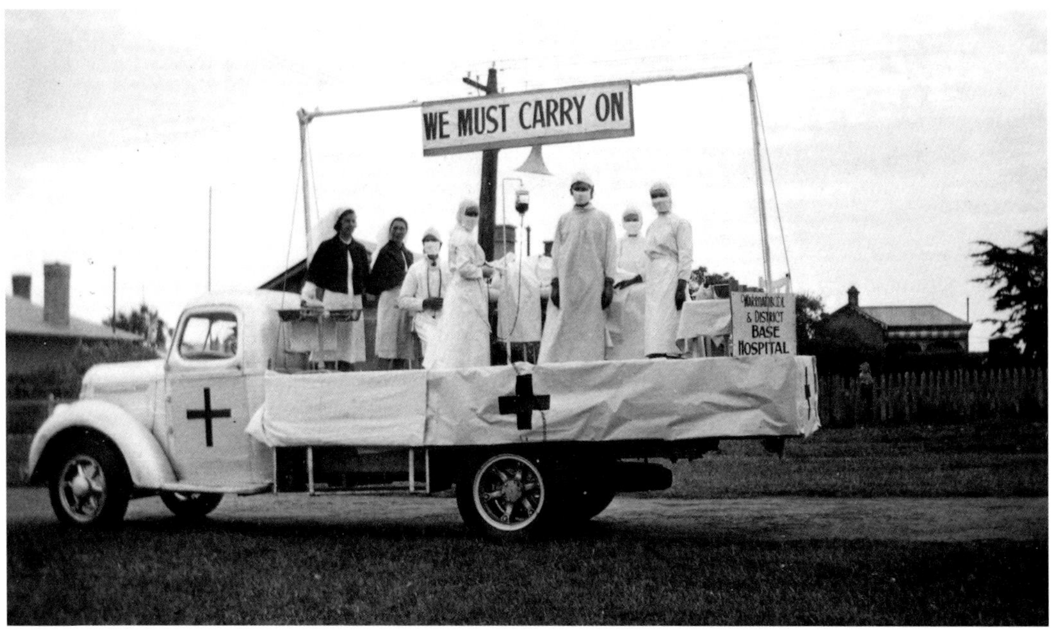

Hospital float, street parade, 1937

to cut, stack, load and cart the wood. Each district tried to outdo the others in the amount of wood cut and stacked, as shown in headlines in the *Standard* on successive weekends in March and April 1930: "Splendid achievement at Panmure—91 tons stacked"; "Nullawarre North gets busy—more than 90 tons cut"; "Record wood chop—Nirranda's Splendid Effort—104 tons cut and stacked".

Many more examples could be given to illustrate the extent of community involvement in the Warrnambool Hospital which developed during the 1920s and 1930s. This community involvement was an important factor in enabling the Hospital to make the transition from a charity benevolent asylum run primarily for the aged poor by a small circle of Warrnambool's elite, to a modern base hospital offering health care to the all people in the town and the district. One of the major barriers to developing a modern hospital was the different scale of funding required, and the involvement of the whole community in working for the Hospital was an essential step to widening the institution's financial base.

[1] Committee of Management Minutes, 28 December 1905.
[2] Committee of Management Minutes, 5 January 1912.
[3] *Standard,* 9 September 1926.
[4] *Standard,* 27 September 1926.
[5] For the development of other hospital auxiliaries, see Peter Yule, *The Royal Children's Hospital: A History of Faith, Science and Love,* Melbourne, 1999, ch.6.
[6] Mrs N. Moore, "Warrnambool Base Hospital Senior Ladies Auxiliary: 1923–1996", unpublished typescript in WBHA.
[7] *Standard,* 31 January 1928.
[8] *Standard,* 31 January 1928.

Chapter 8

DOCTORS AND DISEASES

At the meeting of the Warrnambool Hospital committee of management in January 1902 Mr Parrington gave notice that he would move, "That in the opinion of the committee it is desirable for the more efficient and more economical management of the Hospital that the services of a Resident Medical Officer be engaged." Although the motion was passed and reaffirmed at subsequent meetings, there was considerable opposition, primarily on the grounds that it was a mistake to replace an experienced part time paid medical officer with an inexperienced doctor straight out of medical school. Partly as a result of this opposition and partly from difficulty in obtaining a suitable doctor, it was not until May 1903 that Dr Reginald Howden became the Hospital's first resident.

It is difficult to explain why the Warrnambool Hospital did not employ resident doctors until shortly before its golden jubilee, as most hospitals of the era found the cheap labour of junior resident doctors the only way to care for large numbers of patients at an affordable cost. However, Warrnambool persisted with the employment of an experienced doctor as part time paid medical officer, possibly a reflection of the low numbers of patients, or else of loyalty to local doctors. By the turn of the century, however, a majority of the committee came to realise that the Hospital could no longer function efficiently with a part time medical officer. In addition, it seems that the long-standing friction between the paid medical officer and the Hospital's honoraries led to the honoraries supporting the appointment of a junior doctor as resident. The main grievance of the honoraries was that the paid medical officer had exclusive right to perform all operations at the Hospital and, in contrast to most other hospitals, the honoraries were not given control of beds, this being the prerogative of the paid medical officer.[1] The change in the balance of power in favour of the honoraries was reflected in the rules adopted for the resident medical officer:[2]

1. The RMO should reside on the premises and not leave for more than four hours without calling in an honorary medical officer as replacement.
2. The RMO should not be absent for more than 24 hours without obtaining the consent of the president.
3. The RMO shall not engage in private practice.
4. The RMO shall be under the direction of the honorary medical officers.
5. The RMO shall visit the wards of the institution at least twice daily.

6. The RMO shall supervise the master, the nursing staff and all the servants and inmates and in case of neglect of duty shall suspend any of them and report to the committee.
7. Each patient shall be allotted to an honorary medical officer on admission (except for the paying patients who could choose their doctor) and shall be in the charge of that doctor until discharge.
8. The RMO shall perform no major operations without consultation with at least one honorary medical officer.

The exclusive right of the paid medical officer to perform operations was removed and from this time almost all operations at the Hospital were performed by the honorary medical officers.

We know little of Dr Reginald Howden, the first resident medical officer at the Warrnambool Hospital, except that he was a graduate of the University of Melbourne and that he gave satisfactory service for twelve months before returning to Melbourne. His monthly reports to the committee show that he had a genuine concern for the well-being of his patients, but of his professional competence and later career we are ignorant.

We know more about his successor. Percy Brett was born in 1879, the son of the Sheriff of Beechworth, and educated at Geelong College and the University of Melbourne. He graduated in medicine in 1904, and soon after was appointed resident medical officer at the Warrnambool Base Hospital. After nine months in Warrnambool he gained an appointment at the Children's Hospital in Melbourne, where he stayed for nearly three years. He entered general practice in Hawthorn and Toorak and gradually began to specialise in obstetrics and gynaecology, being on the honorary staff of the Women's Hospital for many years. A colleague wrote of him that, "His disposition appeared sober and serious, and although not pessimistic, he was continually beset by worries and anxieties." He lacked brilliance but compensated with diligence. Percy Brett died in Melbourne in 1968.[3]

Although the resident medical officers were appointed for a twelve month term, before 1914 not one resident appears to have served a full term, with the actual length of stay averaging about four months. This indicates that the position of resident medical officer at Warrnambool was not a highly desirable post for a young doctor. In those days many aspiring general practitioners went straight into private practice after finishing their degrees, while those who aspired to specialist status sought resident positions at the Melbourne teaching hospitals. It seems that those who came to Warrnambool were generally waiting for an opening in private practice and left as soon as one came up. The only known exceptions to this were Percy Brett, Philip Parer and Edward Rowden White, who all received positions on the resident staff of the Children's Hospital. Edward Rowden White (brother of the well-known physician and philanthropist, Alfred Edward Rowden White) was the only pre-war resident at the Warrnambool Hospital to rise to the heights of the medical profession in Melbourne, becoming a leading consultant at the Women's Hospital before dying as a prisoner of war in Malaya.

It is interesting, given the difficulties that the Hospital had in attracting and keeping residents, that the Hospital had only one woman resident doctor before the Second World War. In the early 1900s increasing numbers of women were graduating from the University of Melbourne Medical School, but most found it very hard to find resident positions.[4] In spite of the large number of women seeking resident appointments, the Warrnambool Hospital only employed one woman, Dr Alice McLean, and her appointment was temporary, lasting only a month before she was replaced by a man. The issue of employing women doctors seems never to have been debated by the committee of management; it was just assumed that a doctor should be a man.

Although there was a rapid turnover of resident doctors in the years before 1914, there had only been brief intervals when the Hospital was without a resident. However, this changed during the First World War when it became almost impossible for country hospitals to obtain resident doctors, as virtually all male graduates joined the armed forces leaving the women to fill the positions at the major Melbourne hospitals. At Warrnambool, Dr Lionel Davy remained as resident until October 1914, but the Hospital was unable to obtain a successor. With the exception of a short period in mid-1915, the Hospital had to function without a resident doctor until 1920. As several of the honorary doctors were also absent at the war, the workload for the remaining honoraries must have been enormous, especially during the influenza epidemic of 1919.

In the 1920s the Hospital was able to obtain resident doctors on a more regular basis than before the war, with most staying in Warrnambool for at least twelve months. Most residents of the time used their hospital position as training for general practice, although only one, Dr Alf Brauer, chose to remain in Warrnambool. Dr Brauer became one of the most respected doctors in Warrnambool. We know relatively little about most of the other residents, but it would be interesting to know more about the eloquently named Dr Wesley George Catchlove Godbehear, resident in 1923–24.

By the end of the 1920s the Hospital had become accustomed to having a regular supply of resident medical officers, and some consideration was being given to employing a second resident to cope with the continually rising number of patients. However, throughout the first half of the 1930s it again became very difficult to obtain the services of a resident, and for long periods of time the Hospital had to manage without one. There was a general shortage of junior doctors at the time as the Depression made it impossible for many families to support their children through the lengthy medical course. Once again the burden of the day to day routine of patient care fell on the honoraries, who appear to have carried the extra load with little complaint.

The years 1900 to 1939 were the heyday of the general practitioner honorary at the Warrnambool Hospital. At the start of the period the senior part time medical officer was replaced by the junior resident medical

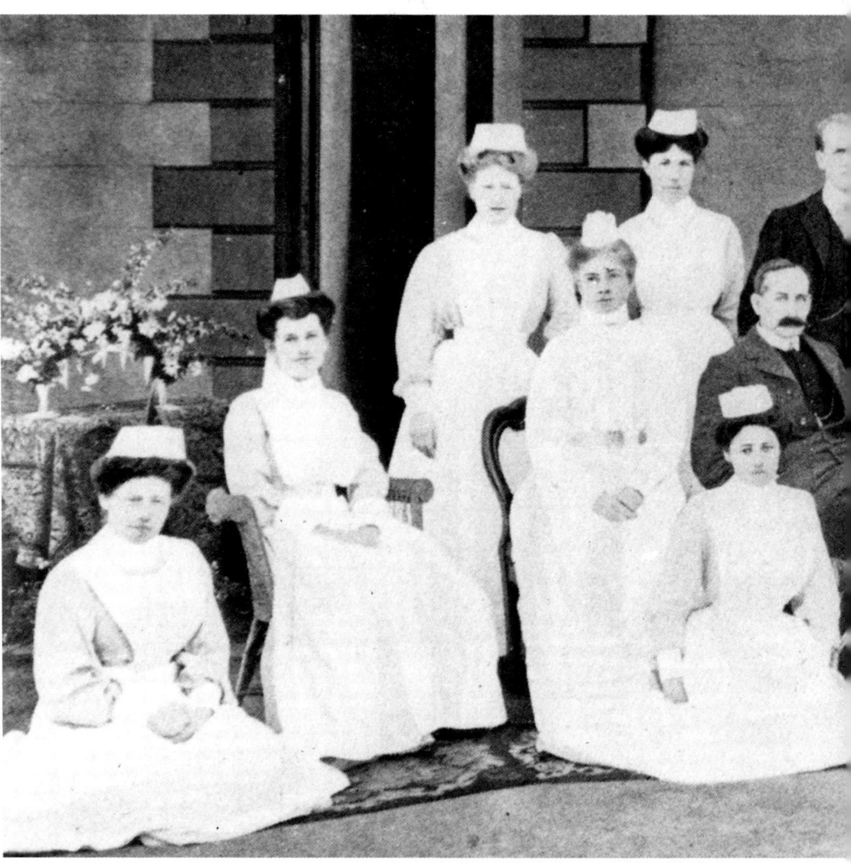

officer, and control of beds and the right to operate were given to the honorary medical officers. At the end of the period, the Hospital was beginning to take the first steps toward the employment of specialists, which, over the next fifty years were to lead to the gradual diminution of the role of the town's general practitioners in the work of the Hospital.

The more active role taken by the honorary staff after the turn of the century led to the decision to follow the example of most metropolitan hospitals and introduce a degree of specialisation among the honoraries. The honorary appointments were divided between surgical and medical, with senior doctors receiving inpatient appointments, while the more junior doctors attended the outpatient clinics. However, the new arrangement does not seem to have greatly affected the actual functioning of the Hospital, with some of the honorary physicians regularly performing surgery and the honorary surgeons attending patients with purely medical conditions.

At the turn of the century Drs Thomas Scott and Thomas Fleetwood were approaching retirement and a new generation of doctors was beginning to take over their role as the mainstays of the honorary staff of the Hospital. The most prominent of these were Charles Macknight, Horace Holmes,

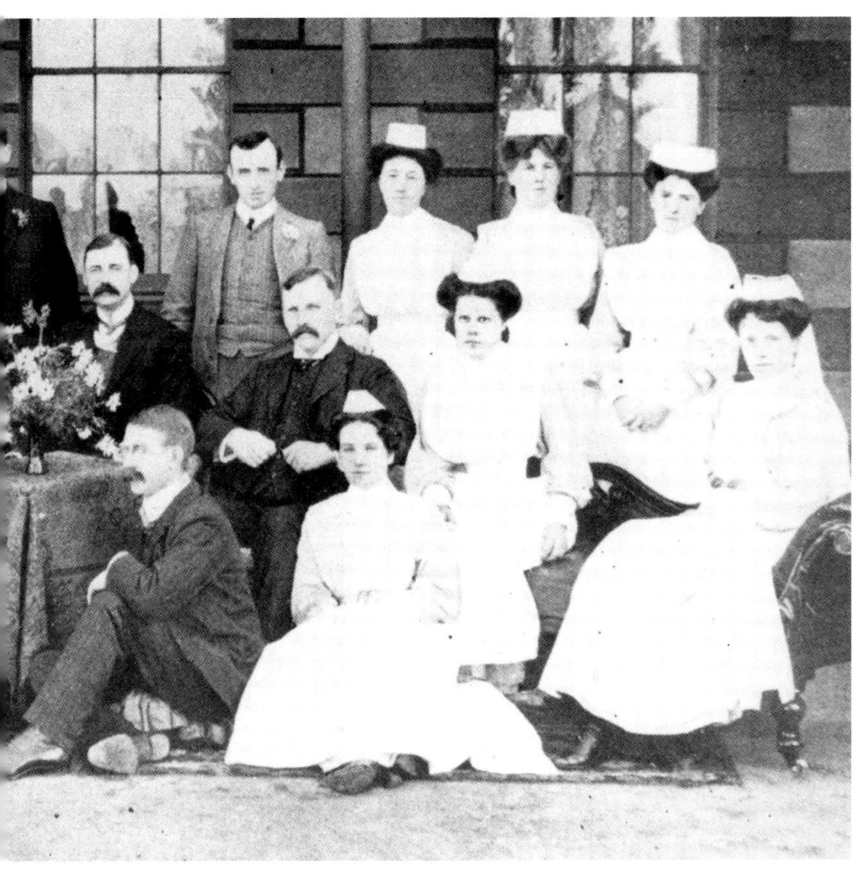

Hospital staff, 1908

John Hunter Henderson, F.E. Littlewood, and Egbert Connell and these men dominated the Warrnambool medical world in the years before the Second World War.

Dr Charles Macknight was the son of Charles Macknight, a Scottish squatter who settled at "Dunmore", between Hawkesdale and Macarthur, in the early 1840s. Dr Macknight was educated at Melbourne Grammar School and the University of Edinburgh before commencing practice at "Dunmore" in Koroit Street (now the offices of Coffey, Hunt and Co.) in the 1890s. Except for service overseas in the First World War, Dr Macknight spent his entire career in Warrnambool and, as Dr Littlewood recalled, he "took a personal interest in the lives of his patients and was conversant with the pedigree and family history of nearly all of them". He never aspired to surgery, but was considered the leading physician on the Hospital's honorary staff and, later in his career he increasingly specialised in anaesthetics and "was cheerfully on call at any hour of the day or night".[5]

"I, Horace Iles Holmes, M.D., F.R.A.C.S., came to Warrnambool on November 15th, 1905 to take over the practice of Thomas Faulkner Fleetwood, F.R.C.S. Ireland etc." With these words, Dr Horace Holmes began his account of the medical history of Warrnambool.[6] Dr Holmes was born in Tasmania in 1877 and studied medicine at the University of Melbourne (after his initial studies at the University of Tasmania were interrupted by an attack of typhoid fever.) He graduated in the top six of his year, an achievement which was rewarded by an appointment as resident at the Melbourne Hospital, and he also served as a resident at Launceston and the Women's Hospital. As shown by his M.D., F.R.A.C.S., he had senior qualifications in both medicine and surgery, but it was as the leading surgeon on the honorary staff for many years that he made his greatest contributions to the Warrnambool Hospital. He recalled that the operating theatre when he arrived "was a single room with a concrete floor, an outside door, and a skylight or lantern into which in hot weather blow flies used to gather and buzz until tired". Although Dr Holmes' interest at the Hospital was primarily surgical, in private practice he was, like all his colleagues, a general practitioner. He sold his practice to Dr C.B. Berryman in 1944 and died in 1959.

Dr John Hunter Henderson was, like Charles Macknight, a graduate of the University of Edinburgh and he also obtained his fellowship of the Royal College of Surgeons. He came to Australia in the early 1900s and purchased the practice of Dr J.W. O'Brien in Warrnambool in 1904. This practice was located at "Ellerslie House" in Koroit Street and later moved across the road to a surgery previously occupied by Dr J. Grattan Wilson. Dr Henderson shared much of the surgical load at the Hospital with Dr Holmes, and was heavily involved as a committee member for many years.

Dr Frank Littlewood worked as a locum in both Koroit and Warrnambool before purchasing the practices of Drs Craig and Baldwin in 1915. He moved these practices to Kepler Street opposite the Masonic Hall and was a popular general practitioner until his retirement in 1946. Dr Littlewood made an important contribution to the work of the Hospital for many years, particularly on the surgical side.

Dr Egbert Connell graduated from the University of Melbourne in 1892 and in 1899 he succeeded Dr S.V. Theed in a practice in Koroit Street opposite the Baptist Church. He remained there until his death from pneumonia in 1928, when the practice was sold to Dr Alf Brauer. Dr Connell took an active part in hospital work, both as physician and surgeon, and frequently acted as spokesman for the honorary medical officers.

This group of doctors, and their colleagues who did not spend their entire careers in Warrnambool, were all general practitioners. Even though some, such as Horace Holmes, had specialist qualifications, they made their livings as family doctors and in both their hospital and private work they dealt with the whole range of medical and surgical problems. In the inter-war years, however, several younger doctors came to Warrnambool who can be seen as the forerunners of the specialists of today, notably Drs James Patrick and Irving Buzzard.

Dr Patrick graduated from the University of Melbourne in 1912 and, after war service, came to Warrnambool in 1919, when he commenced practice in Liebig Street opposite the library. Dr Patrick ran a general practice, as well as being an honorary surgeon to the Hospital, and is remembered as "a quiet, unassuming and very kind gentleman".[7] At that time the Hospital had no x-ray plant, although most of the general practitioners had their own (very basic) x-ray equipment, and, as Dr John Barnaby, the resident, reported to the committee in 1925:

> At the present time, cases requiring x-ray examination have to be taken away to the Honoraries' own rooms. This means that very sick people cannot be examined as they should be, and also treatment must fall short of the standard required at the present time. Might I recommend the purchase of a plant?[8]

The committee probably did not need a junior resident to tell it that a hospital without x-ray equipment in the mid-1920s was behind the times, and a new x-ray plant was included in the building programme of the late 1920s. At this time each honorary was theoretically responsible for his own radiological work, but Dr Patrick showed the most interest in radiology and he became the Hospital's *de facto* radiologist, a position which was formalised in the following decade. At the annual meeting of the Hospital in August 1937, the committee reported that "the question of specialisation has been discussed very fully and a commencement in this direction will be inaugurated shortly . . . adding to the existing prestige of your base hospital." Several weeks later the *Standard* reported:

> At a commencement fee of £800 per annum, Dr Patrick was last night appointed by the committee of the Base Hospital as radiologist to the institution, his appointment to date from Monday next. Dr Patrick . . . has disposed of his practice in Liebig-street . . . Cr Philpott said that the appointment would make this district an important one in specialised hospital work . . . In his application, Dr Patrick drew attention to the need for improved facilities and equipment in the X-ray room, and Dr. Henderson said that a dressing-room, a room for private patients, and an office would be required.[9]

The senior nature of Dr Patrick's appointment is suggested by his rate of pay, which was eight times the level of a resident doctor's. He held the position of radiologist at the Hospital until his retirement in 1946 and did a great deal, not only to develop radiology at the Hospital, but also to demonstrate the value of specialist appointments.

While Dr Patrick was the only senior specialist appointed to the staff of the Warrnambool Hospital before the Second World War, other new doctors brought specialist skills to the town, even if they worked in general practice. Dr Irving Buzzard came to Warrnambool in 1928, succeeding to the practice built up by Drs Moreton, Makin and Dunstan on the corner of Liebig Street, Raglan Parade and Darling Street. Dr Buzzard's arrival coincided with the opening of the Hospital's first maternity ward, and he quickly built up a reputation as the town's leading obstetrician. With the sole exception of Horace Holmes, Dr Buzzard was the only Warrnambool doctor of the inter-war years to publish in the professional journals, and his reports of unusual cases appeared regularly in the *Medical Journal of Australia*. Many stories are still told in Warrnambool of his skill and he can be regarded as the town's first specialist in obstetrics and gynaecology.

In July 1939 Dr Buzzard published a paper, "Pre-eclamptic toxaemia" in which he discussed the causes, pathology, clinical course and treatment of this dangerous complication of pregnancy.[10] Preeclamptic toxaemia is characterised by a rise in blood pressure, oedema, and albumin in the urine and can have serious consequences for both mother and baby, with the possibility of the mother developing eclampsia (fits, convulsions and coma), chronic nephritis and hypertension, while the baby frequently dies *in utero*. Dr Buzzard based his article on 1,197 patients he had attended in Warrnambool in the previous ten years. One of these was:

> Mrs M., aged twenty-eight years [and] expected to be confined on December 7 1933. Her first pregnancy had been perfectly normal twenty months previously. On October 3, 1933 (thirty-first week of pregnancy), in the course of an antenatal examination I found [hypertension, oedema and raised albumin levels]. I admitted her to hospital, and for the next four weeks [her blood pressure and albumin levels gradually rose]. Medicinal stimulation was tried four times without success. Rupture of the membranes was finally carried out in conjunction with stimulating treatment on December 4 and a living baby was delivered. During this period results of the patient's kidney function tests never departed from the normal.
>
> This patient now has a chronic nephritis. She may have had an underlying nephritis beforehand, and pregnancy, that certain test of kidney function, may have caused it to light up . . . I have advised the patient against subsequent pregnancies, and *post hoc* or *propter hoc* her husband left her soon after the birth of the child.

Dr Buzzard argued that careful monitoring of the patient's condition and careful attention to diet were the basis for treating a mother with preeclamptic toxaemia and he noted that only one of his patients in Warrnambool had developed eclampsia. This paper attracted favourable reviews and was considered to be the definitive statement on preeclamptic toxaemia at the time.

It was not only through the medical journals that Warrnambool's doctors remained in touch with the wider medical world. In 1901 the committee minutes noted that the Hospital's medical officer, Dr Moreton, was organising a local branch of the British Medical Association.[11] Later Dr Holmes was the inaugural president of the Western District subdivision of the Victorian branch of the B.M.A. A regular feature of medical life in the inter-war years were meetings of the Victorian branch at the Warrnambool Hospital. These meetings were attended by many of Melbourne's leading doctors and were not just social events (though the social aspect was not unimportant), but included major clinical meetings with presentations by both Warrnambool and visiting doctors. The meeting held at the Hospital on 22 July 1933 was typical of these.[12] Visiting doctors included Professor

Marshall Allan, Drs Geoffrey Penington, Alfred Coates, Montefiore Silberberg[13], Stewart Cowen, Colin Macdonald, Lesley Hurley and Victor Hurley, all leaders in their fields. Most members of the honorary staff of the Warrnambool Hospital made presentations; among others Horace Holmes discussed cases of toxic thyroid adenoma, carbuncle of the kidney, and exophthalmic goitre, Alf Brauer showed a patient with intestinal obstruction caused by Meckel's diverticulum and another with Paget's disease, Edward Bannon discussed a case of lymphatic leukaemia and Irving Buzzard showed a thirteen year old boy with endocarditis. The visiting doctors contributed extensively to the discussion of the cases and the Warrnambool doctors acknowledged the usefulness of this in keeping them up to date with the latest medical developments.

Although the Warrnambool Hospital was fortunate in the calibre of the honorary staff in the years 1900 to 1939, and there was a steady improvement in the facilities and equipment available for the care of patients, the medical staff were continually faced with patients suffering from diseases for which they could offer no better treatments than their nineteenth century predecessors. The understanding of disease processes improved greatly in the early twentieth century, but with the exception only of the introduction of salvarsan in 1911, insulin in 1921 and, at the very end of the period, of the first of the sulpha drugs, there were very few genuine advancements in treatments. The doctors of 1939 could do nothing for the many cases they saw of overwhelming infections and many people still died or were disabled by diseases such as tuberculosis, osteomyelitis, rheumatic fever, diphtheria and other conditions which are rarely encountered today.

[1] See, for example, *Standard*, 3 February 1893 for a clear statement of the grievances of the honorary doctors.

[2] Committee of Management Minutes, May 1902.

[3] *Medical Journal of Australia*, 1 February 1969.

[4] Before 1914 the Melbourne Hospital took the top six graduates as residents regardless of sex, but almost all other hospitals showed a great preference for men, regardless of ability.

[5] Dr F.E. Littlewood, "Charles Crawford Macknight", obituary in *Medical Journal of Australia*, 23 January 1954, p.146.

[6] Copies of Horace Homes unpublished and untitled memoir are in WBHA and the Warrnambool Public Library.

[7] Interview with Mrs Mirth Jamieson (nèe Marfell), 7 April 1999.

[8] Resident Medical Officer's Report Book, WBHA, 31 July 1925.

[9] *Standard*, 14 October 1937.

[10] Irving Buzzard, "Preeclamptic Toxaemia", *Medical Journal of Australia*, 8 July 1939, pp.55–58.

[11] For many decades the Australian medical profession enjoyed the advantages of their professional association being a branch of a larger international organisation and Australian doctors were members of the British Medical Association.

[12] This meeting was reported in the *Medical Journal of Australia*, 23 and 30 December 1933.

[13] Dr Montefiore Silberberg was the leading cardiologist in Melbourne. He had strong Western District connections as he was the son of a Jewish storekeeper in Branxholme.

Chapter 9

PATIENTS AND THEIR ILLNESSES, 1900–1939

Margaret Emily McCullough and William Maloney were married in 1904 and set up their home in Nicol Street (now Hyland Street). Over the next twenty-five years they had thirteen children, the older ones being born at home, while the younger ones were born at a private hospital in Merri Crescent. Unusually for the time, all the Maloney children survived childhood, but not without some of them being hospitalised with some of the serious childhood illnesses common in the early twentieth century. Peggy was one of the many children in Warrnambool to catch diphtheria in the 1920s and was sent to the isolation ward. Although she knew some of the other children in the ward, she was allowed no visitors and had no contact with her family for the three weeks she was there. She was treated with diphtheria anti-toxin and recovered fairly quickly. Peggy's younger sister, Nell, also developed diphtheria and spent time in the isolation ward. Her brother, Arthur, recalls that their eldest sister, Beth, used to pass food for the two girls over the back fence of the isolation ward.[1]

The third youngest Maloney child, Norma, suffered for many years from chronic ear aches. This was very common among children in the pre-antibiotic era. Little could be done to ease the severe pain, although a sock filled with salt and heated in the oven provided some relief when held over the sore ear. In 1934 Dr Littlewood, the Maloney family doctor, and an honorary surgeon at the Hospital, decided to perform a mastoidectomy. This was a very common operation in the 1930s, but Norma's condition must have been particularly bad as Dr Littlewood did not do a standard cortical mastoidectomy, but a radical mastoidectomy, in which the mastoid antrum and the middle ear are made into one continuous cavity for drainage of infection. This procedure inevitably causes hearing loss, and Norma has been deaf in one ear ever since. The doctor told her that the chloroform anaesthetic would smell nice and give her pretty dreams, but it was horrid and she had nightmares afterwards. The days after the operation were very stressful for the Maloney family as the doctors could not tell if the infection had been fully removed. Norma was in the new children's ward and she remembers that the plates in the ward had the alphabet around the edges and the children learnt to recite the alphabet backwards. During her stay, a well-meaning orderly offered to take Norma to see the little hammer and chisel the surgeon used to cut through her skull, but she was horrified at the idea. After three weeks Norma went home for a long convalescence. She recalls her father giving her a treat by taking her on his Sunday buggy ride and telling a friend that she was "the one we nearly lost".

In the mid-1930s the Maloney family was struck by tragedy when Beth's husband, Baden Wines, developed a brain tumour. Neurosurgery was in its infancy, and, although Dr Littlewood attempted surgery, it was unsuccessful and Baden's condition rapidly worsened. Baden was in great pain from the pressure of the tumour and Dr Littlewood used leeches to relieve the pressure. Arthur recalls going to Boggy Creek with his brothers to collect leeches and Norma still remembers her horror on visiting Baden and seeing the leeches clinging to his head. Baden died in 1936 leaving Beth with two young children.

Arthur Maloney was hospitalised with appendicitis in 1939. By this time appendectomies had become a routine procedure and there were no complications. Arthur had a small crystal set and he remembers that many people crowded around his bed on 4 September to listen to Mr Menzies' announcement that Australia was at war with Germany. Coincidentally, Arthur was also in the Hospital the day the War ended, recovering from malaria he had contracted in New Guinea.

The care given to the Maloney children is indicative of many of the changes which occurred at the Warrnambool in the early years of the twentieth century. The family was typical of the majority of Warrnambool families in that they would have been ineligible for treatment under the old charity hospital rules, but would probably not have been able to afford private hospital treatment. The more flexible admissions policies adopted in the early 1900s enabled the Maloneys and many other families to receive affordable treatment at the Warrnambool Hospital. Peggy and Nell were treated in the infectious diseases ward, which had always been open to anyone of any age with a notifiable infectious disease, but until the opening of some beds for children in the early 1920s, the Hospital actually had a rule prohibiting the treatment of children as inpatients on the grounds that they should not be placed in the same ward as adults. Norma Maloney was among the first generation of children to be treated in the children's ward.

One of the most fascinating records in the Hospital archives is the Resident Medical Officers' Report Book, 1907 to 1927. In this book the resident made a report of the numbers of patients admitted, treated, and discharged each month, the number of operations performed, and the names, ages and causes of death of all those who died in the Hospital in the month. This book thus provides a vivid insight into the changing patterns of disease, the impact of epidemics on the town and district and even some insight into the characters of the residents themselves, with some being bold enough to lecture the committee on the running of the Hospital, while others were so unsure of themselves that they listed three possible causes of death for each patient who died.

The residents' report book is not entirely reliable as a source of statistics. Different doctors used different names for the same disease. Phthisis for tuberculosis, and summer diarrhoea, infantile diarrhoea, enterocolitis or colitis for the childhood gastroenteritis that killed many babies in the early twentieth century are two examples.

In addition, the reports were often incomplete during the war years

CAUSES OF DEATH LISTED IN RESIDENTS' REPORT BOOK, 1907–1927

Cause	No.
Abortion (an 18 year old in March 1921)	1
Abscess of liver	2
Abscess of neck	1
Accident	16
Addison's disease	1
Albuminuria of pregnancy	1
Anaemia	13
Apoplexy	1
Appendicitis	19
Ascites	1
Asthma	1
Brain abscess	1
Bright's disease	3
Bronchitis	6
Burns	5
Caesarean section	2
Cancer – abdominal	2
Cancer – bone	1
Cancer – bowel	1
Cancer – brain tumour	4
Cancer – breast	1
Cancer – colon	6
Cancer – gastric carcinoma	3
Cancer – larynx	1
Cancer – liver	6
Cancer – lung	2
Cancer – melanoma	1
Cancer – oesophagus	2
Cancer – pancreas	2
Cancer – prostate	6
Cancer – rectum	1
Cancer – stomach	6
Cancer – testes	1
Cancer – tongue	1
Cancer – uterus	6
Cancer	13
Cellulitis	1
Cerebral abscess	4
Cerebral haemorrhage	14
Cerebral oedema	1
Cerebral thrombosis	2
Choleycystitis	1
Chorea	1
Chronic alcoholism	3
Cirrhosis of liver	6
Cleft palate	1
Colitis	1
Compound fracture	1
Congenital debility	1
Copraemia	1
Cystitis	4
Delirium tremens	1
Diabetes	5
Diarrhoea	1
Diphtheria (note epidemic September 1916–mid-1918)	38
Dropsy	1
Duodenal ulcer	1
Dysentery	1
Eclampsia	2
Emphysema	1
Encephalitis lethargia (Sept and Oct 1920)	3
Encephalitis	1
Enlarged prostate	7
Epithelioma	3
Erysipelas	1
Gangrene	1
Gastric ulcer	2
Gastritis	1

when the Hospital rarely had a resident doctor. Nonetheless, the reports give an accurate picture of the main causes of death and, while the deaths from old age, cancer and heart disease are little different from today, the reports show the large numbers of deaths that used to occur from diphtheria, tuberculosis, tetanus, and many other diseases that are now extremely rare.

Cause	Number
Gastro-colic fistula	1
Gastroenteritis (inc infantile diarrhoea)	21
General debility	1
Goitre	2
Gun shot wounds	1
Haematemesis	1
Haemorrhage neonatorum	1
Haemorrhage	1
Heart disease	82
Hemiparesis	1
Hemiplegia	4
Hepatitis	1
Hydatids	2
Hydrothorax	1
Ileocolitis	1
Infected ulcer	1
Influenza (none listed till May 1919)	16
Intestinal obstruction	6
Intussusception	3
Laryngitis	2
Leukaemia	1
Locomotor ataxia	1
Lung abscess	2
Malnutrition	5
Marasmus	1
Measles	1
Meningitis	4
Miscarriage	1
Myelitis	1
Nephritis	39
Oedema of larynx	1
Osteomalacia	1
Otitis media	2
Pancreatitis	1

Cause	Number
Paralysis agitans	1
Paralysis	1
Paraplegia	1
Parturition	1
Perforated bowel	1
Perforated duodenal ulcer	1
Peritonitis	4
Pneumonia (includes broncho-pneumonia)	69
Polioencephalitis	1
Polycystic kidneys	1
Prematurity	4
Prostratitis	2
Puerperal sepsis	1
Pulmonary abscess	1
Pyaemia	2
Pyelitis	1
Pyloric stenosis	1
Raynaud's disease	1
Renal failure	1
Rheumatic fever	5
Rodent ulcer	1
Ruptured bladder	1
Salpingitis	1
Senility	100
Septic meningitis	1
Septic pharyngitis	1
Septic phlebitis	1
Septic poisoning	1
Septic thrombosis	1
Septicaemia	8
Spastic paraplegia	1
Stomatitis	1
Suppurating dermoid cyst	1
Syncope	2

Syphilis	1
Tetanus	12
Thrombosis	2
Toxaemia of pregnancy	2
Toxaemia	4
Toxic absorption	1
Tubercular meningitis	8
Tuberculosis	41
Typhoid	12
Uraemia	9
Uterine phlebitis	1
Visceroptosis	1
Whooping cough	1

Age at death:

Age	
less than 1 year	55
1–5 years	54
6–10 years	33
11–20 years	67
21–30 years	66
31–40 years	70
41–50 years	77
51–60 years	102
61–70 years	120
71–80 years	121
81–90 years	61
91–100 years	5
100 years and over	1

In January 1909 the resident reported the death of Thomas Fitzgerald, aged 111, the oldest patient recorded to have died at the Hospital in this period. He would have been born in 1798 or 1799 during the Napoleonic Wars, well before the invention of the railway, and he lived to see the first cars on the road.

One of the most significant features of these figures is the large number who died between the ages of twenty and forty during this period. Some of these were victims of accidents, but a large number died from tuberculosis, complications of pregnancy or from influenza during the epidemic of 1919, which was particularly severe in its impact on young adults.

The First World War and its immediate aftermath saw several major epidemics, some of them worldwide and most of which affected Warrnambool. The first of these was an outbreak of cerebro-spinal meningitis which began at the Broadmeadows army camp in September 1915. Although there was a large army camp at the Warrnambool Racecourse during the war years there is no evidence in the Hospital records of this disease having a major impact in Warrnambool. By contrast, Warrnambool experienced a diphtheria epidemic in 1916–18 at a time when diphtheria was generally on the decline. In September 1916, three children, two five year olds and a two year old, died from diphtheria. These were the first deaths from diphtheria for several years, but they were followed by more during the next two years. Those who died were almost all children under ten. Many more, including Peggy and Nell Maloney, required hospitalisation.

However, the epidemics of cerebro-spinal meningitis and diphtheria were dwarfed by the Spanish influenza epidemic of 1919. This influenza, which caused millions of deaths worldwide, struck Warrnambool in the autumn of 1919. Fortunately there was warning of the approach of the epidemic and the Warrnambool Hospital was able to make some preparations, which included preparing special wards for influenza patients and training "VADs" (Volunteer Aid Detachment—roughly equivalent to nursing aides) to assist the Hospital's nurses. In spite of the preparations, there was very little the Hospital could offer influenza victims except for careful nursing. While Spanish influenza hit all sections of the population, the greatest number of deaths was among young adults. In May 1919, when the epidemic in Warrnambool was at its height, nine influenza patients died in the Warrnambool Hospital with an average age of thirty. This month saw the highest number of deaths in the Hospital in a single month in the Hospital's history up to this time

Although none of the Hospital's nurses died during the influenza epidemic, many became sick and this put great pressure on the Hospital's ability to cope with many very sick patients. Fortunately the community stepped in to help during the crisis and large numbers of volunteers stepped forward to help the nursing staff. It was noted as a great advantage that many women in the town had had first aid training during the First World War and they were able to put this to some use during the influenza epidemic.

The most feared epidemic disease of the first half of the twentieth century was poliomyelitis, or infantile paralysis as it was frequently called. As is often the case, the fear was out of proportion to the actual incidence of the disease; even in epidemic years it was far less common than many other equally dangerous diseases. As with AIDS in recent times, one of the reasons for the reaction to polio was the fear of the unknown. When the first cases were reported in Australia in the early 1900s, doctors had no knowledge of the cause, means of prevention, or treatment of the disease.[2] The first polio epidemic in Melbourne occurred in 1908 and, from the 1920s epidemics became increasingly frequent, with the most serious occurring in 1937–38.

Unfortunately there is little information on the incidence of polio in Warrnambool and district, or of the treatments used at the Warrnambool Hospital. An indication that polio was prevalent in Warrnambool from the very early 1900s is the fact that the Hospital engaged the services of an honorary masseuse in 1904, as massage was the main treatment used for those paralysed by the disease. The epidemics which struck Melbourne in the 1920s do not seem to have attracted as much attention in the Warrnambool district, although Dr Holmes recalled in 1937 that there had been three serious epidemics in the area since his arrival in 1905.[3] However, the 1937–38 epidemic had a major impact, with about twenty-five local cases. In November 1937 the city and shire councils agreed to fund the purchase of a respirator for polio victims who required breathing assistance. The students of the Warrnambool Technical School offered to build a respirator for the Hospital, but the honorary staff appeared to have been doubtful of how good it would be and the offer was refused. Before the summer holidays, Dr Holmes, the city health officer, advised that,

In order to, if possible, prevent infection arriving in Warrnambool . . . all children under 16 years of age arriving in the city should be required to register at the Town Hall. In addition to this he would also recommend that, on registration, a badge to be issued to such child, to be worn in public for a period of three weeks. During that time, no such child would be allowed to enter places of amusement or any place where children were likely to consort.[4]

However, these quarantine efforts were unsuccessful and the disease did reach Warrnambool, with devastating results for those affected. Generally polio patients were treated in the infectious diseases ward of the Hospital for the first three weeks and then received further treatment either in the children's ward or as outpatients, while the most serious cases with long term paralysis were sent to Melbourne for treatment at the Children's Hospital.

It has already been noted that in 1919 the Warrnambool Hospital officially altered its policy and ceased to admit purely benevolent patients, but until the late 1920s the Hospital still had a substantial number of patients who were in the Hospital because they were poor rather than because they were sick. The benevolent patients always provided much of the human interest in the Hospital's officers' reports. In January 1904 the Hospital visitors' report noted:

The House Steward reports that he has taken charge of £2.10.0 belonging to an old age pensioner named Irvine, and he would like the direction of the committee as to whether he can retain it or not. And the Resident Doctor with the House Steward also report that the same patient is a very great nuisance as he leaves the Asylum and returns at his own sweet will, setting the rules of the institution at defiance.[5]

In 1911 the *Standard* reported the death of Mrs Barbara Heath, who had been an inmate of the Warrnambool Benevolent Asylum for twenty-seven years. Mrs Heath was seventy-six and "was an active, loquacious little woman who was well-known to frequent visitors to the institution".[6] A sadder case was that of Henry McDowell, a benevolent patient of "weakening intellect" who wandered away in January 1907 and whose body was found several days later in the Merri River.[7]

The resources freed by the ending of the Hospital's benevolent role went largely to providing treatment to greater numbers of children. Until the early years of the twentieth century, the Hospital had only treated children in emergencies and they were not admitted to the wards. This rule was finally abandoned in 1907 when a "children's corner" was made by placing screens across one end of the male ward. This accommodation was gradually improved and extended in the years up to 1928, when a purpose-built children's ward was opened.

Children have always been victims of a disproportionate number of accidents and accidents filled many of the children's beds. In the early years of the twentieth century many children were injured in accidents involving horses. For example, in 1901 the *Standard* reported that:

A boy named William Riley, aged 13 years, who lives in the east end of the town, met with an accident yesterday. With another boy he had been away getting a load of wood . . . when the vehicle tipped up. Both the lads were thrown to the ground, and Riley fell on his left arm, which was severely injured at the elbow joint. Subsequently he was treated at the Hospital.[8]

William Riley had his arm set by Dr Moreton, but as this was before the opening of the children's corner, he was sent home to convalesce.

Warrnambool's seaside location was the source of many childhood accidents. At a BMA meeting in Warrnambool in May 1939, Dr Edward Bannon,

> showed a boy, aged fifteen years, who had sustained a compound depressed fracture of the right parietal bone, with left hemiplegia. He had been struck by a dislodged stone while at the foot of a cliff, and had been rescued while unconscious by a fireman, who ascended fifty feet of ladders with the boy's inert body strapped across his back.
>
> The boy had been admitted to hospital on June 12, 1938, in a state of unconsciousness; brain tissue was protruding from the wound, and he was completely paralysed on the left side of the body. His eyes deviated to the left. Craniotomy was performed; depressed fragmented bone was removed, pulped brain tissue was swabbed away and the wound was irrigated with acriflavine. A small drain was inserted. The boy was unconscious for a week after the operation. He was given sedatives and magnesium sulphate solution per rectum and nutrient enemata. Dr Bannon said that the boy's eye movement had recovered completely, and he had partly recovered from the hemiplegia.[9]

At the same meeting, Dr Bannon presented the case of,

> a boy, aged 12 years, who on January 18, 1938, had sustained a depressed compound fracture of the frontal bone. The accident had occurred while the boy was fishing; he had fallen and struck his head on a rock. He had walked into the Hospital "to have his head stitched". The frontal bone was trephined and the depressed bone elevated. Recovery was uneventful.

The Hospital treated many children suffering from burns in this period. Open fires, wood-fired stoves, the need to carry hot water for washing, and voluminous clothing for girls all made burn injuries very common. The five deaths from burns recorded in the residents' report book were all of children under eight.

Children were not the only victims of accidents. In May 1937 the *Standard* reported on "a busy day for the ambulance", when Arthur Elliott, the driver of the Warrnambool ambulance attended eight accidents in a single day:

> The first occurred during the morning, when a lady was taken to the Warrnambool Hospital urgently from one of the churches. During the afternoon, his services were required at the racecourse on five occasions, two injured jockeys being subsequently admitted to the Warrnambool Hospital; while in the evening he picked up an aborigine who was knocked down by a car in Liebig-street, and soon after he received another call to the scene of a tragic car accident on the Mailor's Flat road.[10]

At a meeting of the BMA in Warrnambool in May 1939 Dr Edward Bannon presented the case of a 25 year old man who seemed more than usually accident prone. The patient was first admitted to the Hospital on 30 January 1938 "suffering from a lacerated wound of the face, a fracture of the right nasal bone and a fracture of the orbital margin of the right maxilla".[11] He was discharged from hospital on 14 February, but readmitted eight days later with a compound fracture and dislocation of the left elbow joint. He was treated "by means of Kirchner wire extension through the olecranon" and was discharged again on 21 April 1938. This time he remained out of hospital for nine days when he was brought in with a compound depressed fracture of the left frontal bone. Dr Bannon reported that,

> On admission he was deeply unconscious; his temperature was 36.7°C (98°F), his pulse rate was 80 per minute, and his systolic blood pressure was 150 millimetres of mercury. Under light chloroform anaesthesia the wound was extended and a semicircular depressed fracture was revealed. Sound bone was trephined and depressed bone was elevated. Severe haemorrhage occurred. The wound was loosely closed and drainage was provided. The patient remained unconscious for eight days and then gradually recovered. He was discharged, apparently normal, eight weeks; no signs of brain injury was apparent.

The unlucky (or clumsy) patient managed to avoid further injuries up to the time of the meeting, but he did suffer from recurrent frontal headaches.

We are inclined to think that we live in an increasingly violent society, but, while burglaries were rare, the number of victims of gunshot and stab wounds treated in the Warrnambool hospital in the 1920s and thirties suggest that the district was not as quiet as we imagine.[12]

While the reports in the press and the pages of the medical journals give a picture of the dramatic and unusual reasons for admission to the Warrnambool Hospital, it is far harder to find stories of patients admitted with the common diseases of the time. The many people from Warrnambool and district who were treated for tuberculosis, heart disease, cancer, pneumonia, diphtheria, appendicitis, gastroenteritis, typhoid and many other illnesses and the many women who delivered their babies uneventfully after the opening of the maternity ward have left few accounts of their stay. However, the period 1900–1939, and particularly the years between the two world wars, saw a complete change in the public perception of the Hospital. In the nineteenth century the Hospital was seen as a place where the aged poor went to die and only a fairly small proportion of the district's wealthier citizens involved themselves in its work. In the years of Marcus Saltau's presidency the Hospital became the primary deliverer of health care services to the people of Warrnambool and district. The Hospital was opened to all regardless of income and the whole community became involved in supporting it. The quality of treatment rose steadily and the standard of patient care was probably the equal of any hospital outside the major metropolitan teaching hospitals.

[1] Interview with Arthur Maloney, 8 July 1999.
[2] For an account of the unusual epidemiology of polio, see Sir James Spence, *The Purpose and Practice of Medicine,* London, 1960, pp.80–81.
[3] *Standard,* 3 November 1937.
[4] *Standard,* 17 December 1937.
[5] Committee Report Book, 1889–1936, 23 June 1904.
[6] *Standard,* 17 January 1911.
[7] *Standard,* 24 January 1907.
[8] *Standard,* 2 February 1901.
[9] Report of meeting of the Victorian Branch of the British Medical Association in Warrnambool, *Medical Journal of Australia,* 15 July 1939, p.118.
[10] *Standard,* 7 May 1937.
[11] *Medical Journal of Australia,* 15 July 1939, p.118.
[12] See, for example, a report in the *Standard* on 25 May 1935, which talks of "the recent stabbing affray" and reports on the condition of several victims as well as a youth who had been shot in Mortlake.

Chapter 10

NURSING, 1900–1939

Thelma Hance was born in Timaru, New Zealand, in 1905 and came to Australia when she was four. She trained as a nurse at the Warrnambool Hospital in the 1920s and her reminiscences give a vivid picture of the life of a nurse in that era.[1]

> Warrnambool was a town of about 8000 people with approximately six doctors to care for them and I, a young slim girl of eighteen, bursting to begin training as a nurse. The application forms stated one had to be single and aged between twenty-one and thirty years. There was a shortage of applicants. However, after discussions and long consultations with our family doctor (Dr Horace Holmes) I was given permission to apply. So I began a three month probation period without pay—the first eighteen year old applicant and, as I was considered suitable, stayed on. There was no school of nursing, but occasionally the doctors would give us lectures.
>
> Wages had been agreed by the Hospital Board in 1921—£15 annually for the first year; £25 annually in the second year and in our final year £33. We were paid once each calendar month the sum of twenty-five shillings, which worked out to a princely sum of 6/3 a week. Of course, there was not an eight hour day—we usually worked between twelve and fourteen hours a day with no such thing as paid holidays.
>
> Each nurse supplied her own uniform. I needed three uniforms and six aprons plus cuffs, collars and caps to begin with . . .
>
> There were sixteen trainees when I began in 1924 but no Nurses' Home. We slept four in a room in a section between the female ward and outpatients. You can imagine how thrilled we were when the Nurses' Home was opened and we each had our own little room.
>
> How was the Hospital organised? Matron was in charge of everything. There was the Male Ward (Ward 1), Female Ward which also included any children (Ward 2), and Isolation. The Male Ward and Theatre worked in together. Each ward held about twenty-five patients and they were large open wards with beds divided by screens only. There was a sister in Women's Ward with between three and five nurses during the day and a sister in Male Ward with again three to five nurses during the day. At night a senior nurse was responsible for the whole hospital, plus an intermediate nurse in Women's Ward and one junior nurse to help between the two wards. If the senior nurses became concerned about any patient she would call the Matron.

If I was on day duty the junior night nurse would call the day nurses at 6.00 a.m. and we were on duty at 6.30 a.m.

There were no wardsmen so we did everything—nursing, sponging, polishing the floors, cleaning out lockers, doing the flowers, doing pan rounds, sterilising—through to 6.00 p.m. Sometimes we would work from 6.30 a.m. through to 2.00 p.m., be off until 5.00 p.m. then work through till 9.00 p.m. When on day duty we would be given a day off when we could be spared—never a regular day off.

If on night duty we were on for six weeks with no night off. At the end of this period we would be given one sleeping day and one day off.

The junior night nurse was responsible for turning off the lights at 10.30 p.m. All nurses had to be in by 10.00 p.m. We had to sign the book if we went out. We could ask the matron for a late night pass which was occasionally granted—then we could stay out till 11.00 p.m. and very rarely till 11.30 p.m.

Discipline was very strict. Surnames were always used—some of my friends still use my maiden surname. No one would dare use Christian names on duty. Patients were always Mr and Mrs or Miss. Of course a doctor was NEVER called by name.

When my training began I went straight into the Female Ward . . . There was no midwifery at this time—women had their babies in private hospital or at home.

The wards were always full, approximately twenty-five patients in each ward and we were always busy. Patients came in with a variety of fractures. If a hip was broken the person would be bedridden for the remainder of their life. It was only after the Second World War with all the new, advanced technology, that pinning became routine. There were a variety of accidents, some caused by being thrown off horses, out of buggies, and a number of motor bike accidents. In my early days there were few cars and they were certainly not so fast. Female Ward had similar cases as would be seen today. One great difference would be the long stay in bed and constant nursing required, largely because there were none of the modern, fast acting drugs—penicillin, antibiotics etc.

On my first night duty stint there was only a flickering gas jet at one end of the ward and I carried a lantern as I went from bed to bed checking each patient. It was a rather lonely, eerie experience.

Our Isolation Ward always had diphtheria, scarlet fever and polio cases as there was no immunisation against these diseases. I also saw a number of meningitis cases. When we nurses worked in Isolation we slept on the asphalt verandah and stayed in this Ward for about 6 weeks at a time. A person from the Hospital kitchen would bring over our meals, placing them on a wooden bench outside. Then she would ring a bell, and some one from the Isolation kitchen would go out and collect our very plain dinner.

Tuberculosis cases were kept separately and nursed on the verandahs.

When we worked in theatre, which I loved, we were on call twenty-four hours a day Of course equipment was very basic but again we had the full range of cases that would be in a hospital today. All equipment had to be sterilised before we went off duty and the autoclave was *so* slow! I well remember a night when I finished in theatre at 3.00 a.m. and had to be back on duty at 6.00 a.m.

There were few geriatrics in my day—they would be cared for by private nurses in the home or cared for by extended family members. Many of course died earlier, often from a pneumonia complication.

Surgery was similar to today with gall bladders, cancers, colostomies, etc.—but we had no modern, comfortable bags for colostomies, only a dressing and a binder. We always seemed to have a peritonitis patient being drained of pus which required full Fowler's position in bed for about twelve weeks. I often wondered how families coped when mother or father was in hospital for three months or longer.

There were no diuretics so many people came in with dropsy.

We always had sick pneumonias. Every four hours we made large linseed poultices, or sometimes even jackets of linseed, to place on the patient's chest. We nursed and waited for the crisis which came on the eighth day. Then they either collapsed or got better. We were told it was bad nursing if a patient died.

Again I saw a number of tetanus cases but unfortunately they rarely survived. There were also a number of osteomyelitis cases.

Patients in my day had a full sponge every day. There was a pan round after every meal as no one was allowed out of bed. Backs were done every four hours. You would almost be dismissed if a patient got a bed sore.

I well remember the night on duty when we had a boy who had fallen over the cliffs at the beach and hurt his nose. A week later he developed tetanus. He had a little bell and knew to ring it when he was going to spasm. The bell rang when he was at the far end and down I raced. By this time he was black in the face. I was unable to get his padded peg into his mouth, but I managed to get my little finger in where a tooth was missing. The force of his jaws in a spasm was unbelievable. My finger was cut in the process. I had to yell out to a patient who could get out of bed to go and get the nurse on Male Ward. Later matron was called and then another nurse was woken from sleep and came on duty to "special" him. Unfortunately he died a few days later. You can imagine how closely I was watched over the next few days as it was feared I would contract tetanus—of course I kept working!

Apart from all the nursing duties, the junior nurse was responsible for cooking dinner for the night staff. I seem to recall being given few supplies. I can remember sneaking out to the large vegetable garden that was on the south side, where Marcus Saltau now stands, to steal a cabbage to cook to add interest to the meal. You can be sure I took great care to cover up my footprints.

Whenever a death occurred two nurses had to take the body to the mortuary on canvas and poles. Can you imagine two of us trying to hold our lanterns and carrying a heavy body out in the middle of a dark, windy night? Several times the body would be put down on the ground while we caught our breath and invariably, our lanterns went out and we'd have to relight them.

We can all recall funny stories about patients and their difficult behaviours. I remember one old man who at night would yell out, "I'm starving, starving, starving!" The night nurse would reply, "It's alright—we've put a cake in the oven and when it's cooked we'll give you a piece!" It was enough to settle him and off he'd go to sleep. Later during the day he'd start—"I'm dying, dying, dying". The man in the next bed called out, "Well for the love of God, die quiet."

We all enjoyed the fun of helping to raise funds for the Hospital rebuilding on Gala Days.

Of course many patients were in hospital for Christmas and could not be sent home, so we spent our "spare time" decorating the wards with Christmas decorations.

At the end of our training each nurse was presented with a certificate—there were no graduation evenings or gold medal awards.

The reminiscences of Thelma Hance give the modern reader a vivid picture of the life of a nurse at the Warrnambool Hospital in the 1920s. Her training came in the middle of the period 1900 to 1939, a period in which the nurse training school at the Warrnambool Hospital was established and many of the traditions developed which remained strong until the 1980s. Nursing in Warrnambool changed from a very basic and menial job without formal training or recognised qualifications at the end, to being a part of the wider nursing profession with organised training, recognised qualifications and a central, if still very subordinate, place in the health care system.

Nursing staff with resident doctor, 1907

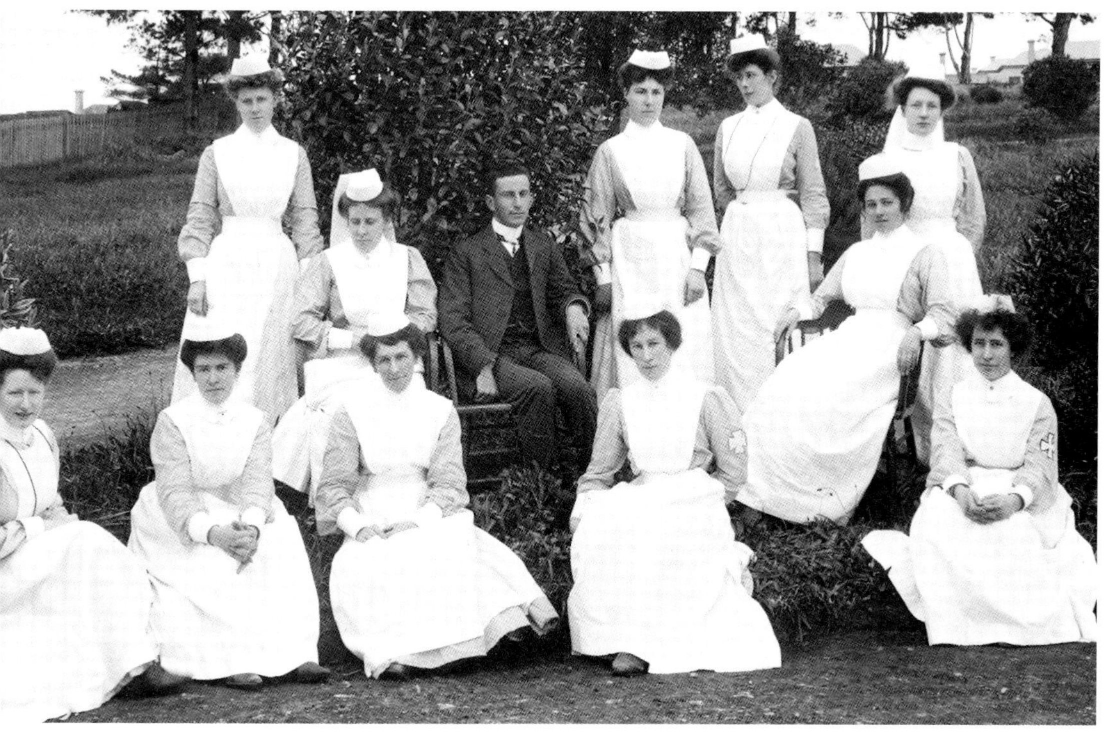

The early part of the period 1900 to 1939 was important in the development of nursing in Warrnambool. The critical step was the decision in 1902 by the committee to affiliate with the Victorian Trained Nurses' Association and have the Hospital placed on the list of recognised training schools for nurses. This meant that the Hospital's trainee nurses for the first time sat for the same exams as nurses at the major Melbourne hospitals, and received widely recognised certificates qualifying them to nurse anywhere in the British Empire. The nurse training course was standardised at three years at this time, with the first trainee to receive the Hospital's certificate being Nurse J.W. Davidson, who later served as matron of the Hospital.

The central feature of the system of nurse training was that it was an apprentice system based on "on the job" training. The trainee nurses worked for three years at a minimal rate of pay and provided a cheap nursing workforce. In return the nurses received a qualification which opened the door to some of the small range of careers open to women at the time—hospital or private nursing, private hospital ownership, and, from the mid-1930s, air hostessing (as early air hostesses required a nursing certificate). The nurses received a small amount of formal theoretical tuition, mainly in the form of lectures by members of the honorary medical staff, the resident doctor or the matron, but almost all their learning was by observing more senior nurses in the wards or by trial and error.

There were four distinct phases in nurse recruitment for the Warrnambool Hospital in the period 1900 to 1939. In the first, from 1900 to 1914, the supply of suitable young ladies seems to have slightly exceeded the demand. In these years the Hospital sought educated and mature women to train as nurses, with the minimum age for entry being raised to twenty in 1906 and twenty-one in 1910 and with a requirement of reasonable literacy and numeracy. The Hospital attempted to ensure that its nurses were "ladies" by insisting that they pay for their own uniforms and work for three months without pay while they were on probation. As it would be extremely difficult for a poor family to afford the uniforms or support an adult daughter for three months, this effectively precluded trainees from poor homes. In spite of these restrictions the Hospital was able to obtain enough trainees to meet its needs from the local area and few nurses came from outside.

During the First World War, the number of aspiring nurses rose sharply as the only way in which girls could serve overseas was as nurses and many felt that it was their patriotic duty to undertake nurse training. Consequently the Hospital was able to be very selective in choosing trainees and the entry regulations were strictly enforced. However, this situation changed very rapidly after the end of the War and, throughout the 1920s, the Hospital had great difficulty recruiting sufficient nurses. The monthly reports by the matrons contain frequent references to this problem. For example, Miss Peacock reported to the committee in December 1922: "A difficulty exists in securing suitable girls to train as nurses; at present I have only three names on my books and not any of these are at all suitable."

The Hospital responded to the shortage of nurses in several ways. As Thelma Hance's story shows, the minimum age for trainees was reduced from twenty-one to eighteen, pay rates were gradually increased and, perhaps most importantly, the Hospital began to look beyond the ranks of "ladies" to find its nurses. In 1921 the Matron, Miss Davidson, told the committee:

> As all the Hospitals are increasing the remuneration for trainees, I am sure that we will have to raise ours considerably—otherwise we will find it impossible to get probationers. Owing to the increased cost of uniforms etc. they need to get much more help from home and in many instances we get our best nurses and noblest girls from homes that are not blessed with much of this world's goods.[2]

The supply and demand situation for nurses again moved sharply with the onset of the Depression in the late 1920s, and for most of the next decade the Hospital had far more applicants than it required. While the entrance requirements were not raised, the Hospital was able to choose the best applicants, while wages and conditions remained unchanged. Rita Brauer came from New South Wales to begin her training in 1927 and recalled that it was difficult to get a position. She came to Warrnambool because a friend of her mother's knew Mr Robertson, the secretary of the Hospital, and she applied through him. Similarly, Wilma Oram remembers that it was very hard to get into nursing in the early 1930s. She came from Murtoa to Warrnambool because she had a connection through the wife of the local rector.

In the years before 1939, trainee nurses did not begin at the Hospital as a group, but individually, or perhaps in pairs as they were required to fill vacancies. Rita Brauer arrived in Warrnambool with another trainee. They were met at the station by Mr Robertson, the Hospital secretary, in a horse-drawn cab and were driven up to the Hospital, where they were treated with some curiosity as having come from out of the district. The new trainees received no preliminary training or induction. On her first day Wilma Oram was assigned to the male ward, where the next most junior nurse took her around and told her what to do. She found that the patients were very helpful to the junior nurses, as many had been in the Hospital a long time and they knew the routine.

All the junior nurses of this period recall their first months at the Hospital as a blur of hard work, exhaustion and rapid learning. There are some differences in recollections of hours of work in the 1920s and 1930s, but nurses on day shift seem to have started work at 6.00 or 6.30 a.m. and worked a twelve hour day, either straight through until about 7.00 p.m., or, in some cases, with a break in the afternoon and then until 9.30 p.m. While on day duty the nurses had one day off each week. Night duty was from 9.00 p.m. until 7.00 a.m. and could be for up to three months without a day off.

Much of the work of the nurses was purely menial, with much cleaning, sweeping, polishing and dusting. Until well into the 1930s there were no taps in the wards and the nurses had to carry water to the wards in buckets. Another task which was well outside the modern definition of nursing duties was stoking the boilers with coal. A boilerman did this during the day, but once he knocked off, the night nurses had to keep the boilers stoked until morning in order to maintain the supply of hot water. The nurses of that era recall that it was very difficult to keep their white aprons clean while shovelling coal. The nurses had to prepare many of the meals for the patients in their wards and serve the meals prepared in the Hospital's kitchens. They also had to sterilise all the ward instruments, cutlery, dishes and so on.

The nurses were gradually introduced to what we regard today as nursing duties. In their first months they would spend much of their time on the personal care of the benevolent and convalescent patients, but by their second year they were given enormous responsibilities for the well-being of their patients. This was particularly so during the lengthy periods in the First World War and the 1930s when the Hospital was without a resident doctor, and quite junior nurses had to decide when it was necessary to call one of the honorary medical staff.

The formal part of a nurse's training was limited to occasional lectures by members of the honorary medical staff, the resident doctor (when there was one) and the matron. Nurses had to attend lectures in their time off work, or if they were on duty, they had to make up the time lost. This could be particularly trying for nurses on night duty. Until 1928 nurses had to go to Melbourne for their exams, but in that year the Hospital was recognised as a nurse training school and was able to hold its own exams. Accreditation could not be granted until the Hospital had a minimum number of beds and this minimum was passed with the opening of the major extensions in 1928.

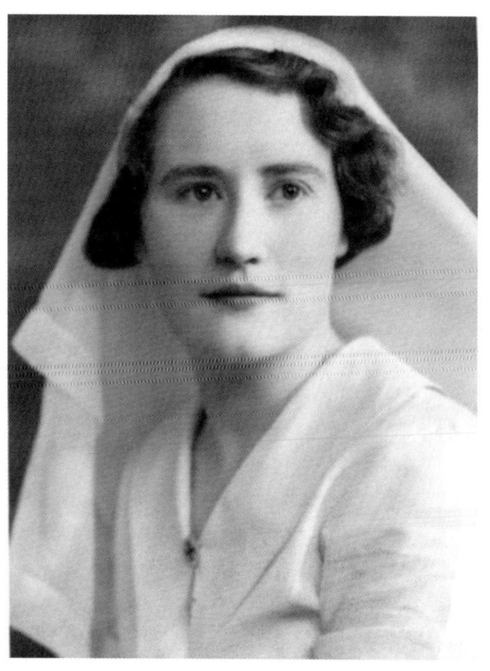
Agnes McNair, 1938

It was often difficult to fit lectures and exams into the busy schedule of the trainee nurses. Wilma Oram recalled that she was nursing in the Isolation Ward when it was time to sit for the surgical exam. The matron sent another nurse over to isolation with the exam paper and instructions to supervise Wilma. However, Dr Bannon, who was to mark the papers, felt that the conditions were unfair for Wilma and he insisted that everyone sit the exam again.

In this era it was not questioned that all nurses should be unmarried and live at the Hospital. Many parents, especially those from out of Warrnambool, would not have allowed their daughters to come nursing if they were not given safe accommodation and had their personal lives strictly monitored. However, until 1924 the living conditions for nurses were very poor. The nurses slept four to a room in a small area near the Female Ward. Thelma Hance recalled that the beds were so close together that the nurses who slept furthest from the door had to climb over the other beds to get to their own. When the new nurses' home was opened in December 1924, all nurses had their own small bedrooms and conditions generally were far more satisfactory. As Matron Lucy Paton reported, "everything is very nice and comfortable and much appreciated."

Nurses in the era 1900 to 1939 were meant to be respectful and obedient to all in authority. Agnes McNair recalled that if the matron or a doctor came into the ward all the nurses, even senior sisters, had to stand to attention with their hands behind their backs. The senior nurses must have found it irksome being "respectful and obedient" to junior resident doctors, but it was accepted at the time that nurses were subordinate to doctors in the health care system.

It is not surprising, given the long hours, hard physical work and close proximity to very sick patients, that many nurses suffered from poor health. This is a recurring theme of the matrons' reports as the nursing staff was frequently disrupted by epidemics of diphtheria, scarlet fever, influenza and other infectious diseases and nurses also had time off with sore throats, septic fingers (so common that it was called "nurses' finger"), and exhaustion. On many occasions, sickness forced nurses to discontinue their training, although there is only one case in this period of a nurse dying from an infectious disease acquired in the Hospital. This was Vida Holmes from Byaduk, who developed poliomyelitis while nursing in the isolation wards during the polio epidemic of 1928, and, in spite of the best efforts of the Hospital's medical and nursing staff, died several months later.

Many nurses did not complete their three years training, leaving because of sickness, marriage or, in many cases, because they did not feel strong enough for the work. The matrons' reports include frequent comments such as: "I am forwarding the resignation of two trainees—Miss McKay on the plea of ill-health. She says she does not feel equal to taking up the work again. Nurse Harkness wishes to be relieved of her duties at once on account of her mother's ill-health."[3] It is not possible to calculate the drop-out rate, but it seems from the matrons' reports that it was probably lower than for the metropolitan hospitals, where it approached thirty per cent in the 1920s.

For many trainee nurses one of the their most arduous experiences was being on duty in the Isolation Wards. The number of nurses allocated to isolation depended on the number of patients, which fluctuated greatly, but for most of the time only one nurse was required. Wilma Oram recalled that she had some time off herself suffering from diphtheria and on her return to duty she was sent to the Isolation Wards. There were four patients at the time, two with diphtheria and two with scarlet fever and they were in separate rooms, a long distance from each other. Wilma was the only nurse and had to care for the patients day and night for twelve weeks. "Old Lizzie" would bring meals over from the kitchen, leave them at the gate and ring the bell so that Wilma would know to collect them. She had to do everything by herself, with the doctor coming every two or three days to check on the patients. Conditions were very bad for the nurses in Isolation, with no proper bedroom nor even a cupboard to hang their clothes. The matrons frequently complained of the poor conditions, but little was done as the Isolation Wards were the responsibility of the city and shire councils rather than the Hospital committee of management.[4]

1928 was an important year in the development of nursing at the Warrnambool Hospital. Not only did the Hospital receive accreditation as a nurse training school, but the number of nurses was increased substantially, from about sixteen to twenty-six, to cater for the increased number of patients, and the opening of the Maternity Ward introduced a major new field for the Hospital's nurses. Miss Nona Griffiths was the matron at this time and she invited Thelma Hance, who had obtained her midwifery qualifications at St George's Hospital in Melbourne, to return to take charge of the maternity ward. For the next five years she was the only sister in the ward and for the first three years she did most of the nursing work herself, only having an extra nurse allocated if the ward was particularly busy or if a patient was very ill.

The Hospital had to have 120 births in a year before it could become a midwifery training school. It passed this figure in the first year, but it was not until 1931 that the midwifery course was formally established with Sister Hance in charge. The first midwifery trainees were Vera Harris from Warrnambool and Ilma Osmond from Port Fairy. The course lasted six months, and Sister Hance recalled that it was worth taking on the extra responsibility to obtain the extra nursing assistance.

Sister Hance was in charge of all maternity cases, both public and private and she remembered that,

> We used to keep patients at least eight to ten days. The private patients had to be full sponged every morning—no getting up to have showers . . . We usually had about twelve mothers and babies. As well as caring for the mothers I helped them handle their new child and cope with breast feeding, bringing the babies to the mothers every three or four hours as needed, as well as closely nursing the little babies, ensuring that they thrived and gained weight.[5]

She frequently had to deliver babies herself if a doctor was delayed or unavailable, and several babies were named after her.

The midwifery course was very popular throughout the 1930s, but it appears that it was abandoned during the war years and never restarted.

The nursing staff was very small in the years before 1939. At the turn of the century the staff consisted of the matron, two sisters and ten nurses. The greatest increases came following the extensions of 1928 and 1937, but there were still only five sisters and thirty nurses at the start of the Second World War in September 1939. In general the nursing staff appears to have been happy and contented, even if in a state of perpetual exhaustion. There appear to have been only two occasions in this period when there was any unrest. In 1906, Matron Lewers resigned when the committee did not support her after she suspended a nurse for "repeated acts of insubordination and disobedience". As the nurse was subsequently asked to resign, along with the new matron, it appears that there might have been more to the case than the committee minutes reveal.[6] In June 1924, the matron, Lucy Paton, reported that "Sisters Stubbs and Neale have sent in their resignations—reasons for same is working under very unsatisfactory conditions and shortage of nursing staff, which meant that the sisters worked very often fourteen to sixteen hours a day." The Hospital responded to this by increasing the number of trainee nurses, but the conditions under which nurses worked only improved very slowly.

The nursing staff in the era 1900 to 1939 was made up primarily of trainees, who stayed at the Hospital for three years, leaving as soon as they had completed their training. The element of continuity and experience was provided by the small number of sisters, who were usually graduates of the Hospital. Until about 1920 the Hospital had only two sisters, one each for the male and female wards, and even in 1939 there were only five. We do not know much about these nurses even though they were obviously vital for the effective running of the Hospital, the proper care of the patients and the successful education of the trainees. An indication of the position they held is given by the comments made by Dr Henderson when Sisters Skinner and Drummond resigned in 1937:

> Dr Henderson expressed regret at the resignation of Sister Skinner and spoke in highly eulogistic terms of the quality of her service both in the theatre and in the ward. She had set a fine example to the nurses and would be greatly missed . . . Keen regret was expressed . . . at the resignation of Sister Drummond, highly eulogistic references being made to her qualities as a Sister, and the wonderful example which she set to members of the nursing staff, the speakers concurring that it was practically impossible to adequately replace her on the staff. It was resolved unanimously that the President and Dr. Henderson interview Sister Drummond and endeavour to retain her services for the Hospital.[7]

Among the other sisters who made important contributions in this period were Margaret O'Brien, Doris Hall and Edna McCormick..

The position of matron at the Warrnambool Hospital was in the midst of transition in the early 1900s. In the nineteenth century the matron was normally a married woman and, for most of the time, the day to day running of the Hospital was in the hands of a husband-wife/master-matron team. The division of responsibilities between the two was never clearly defined, and varied according to the wishes and abilities of the holders of the offices. However, the last married couple to hold the positions of master and matron were the Maxwells and, following their retirement in 1902, the posts were held separately. The position of master began its evolution through various incarnations to emerge eventually as the modern chief executive officer, while the matron gradually began to shed her responsibilities for non-nursing functions. While these developments have a certain look of inevitability today, they did not occur without some difficulties.

In February 1905 the president, Marcus Saltau, pointed out the necessity for defining clearly the duties of the matron and the steward (as the master had recently been renamed) and a sub-committee was appointed to draw up some rules. The following year the sub-committee placed its recommendations before a special meeting of subscribers. The report and the meeting endorsed a very positive statement of the matron's position—she was to be mistress of the household, with authority over the nursing staff and the domestic staff. The sub-committee had recommended that the matron should be subordinate to the resident medical officer, but the meeting did not endorse this, making the matron subordinate only to the committee of management.[8]

The powers of the matron of the Warrnambool Hospital, as determined in 1906, were greater than those of most contemporary matrons. However, although there seem to have been very few conflicts between the matrons and either the committee or the medical staff, the turnover of matrons was very high, with very few staying for more than four years. There were thirteen matrons in the years 1900 to 1939:

Mrs Maxwell	1888–1902
Miss Middleton	1902–04
Miss Lewers	1904–06
Mrs Rose Backhouse	1906–08
Miss E.M. Hooley	1908–14
Miss Reeves	1914–16
Miss Anderson	1916–21
Miss Warrender Davidson	1921–22
Miss Peacock	1922–24
Miss Lucy Paton	1924–26
Miss Jessie McKenzie	1926–27
Miss Griffiths	1927–35
Miss Little	1935–39

Mrs Maxwell was the last of the old-style matrons. Her husband was master of the Hospital and it is unlikely that she had formal nurse training. Her successors, Miss Middleton and Miss Lewers were, by contrast, career nurses who did much to alter the style of nursing at the Warrnambool Hospital from its old-fashioned, virtually pre-Nightingale ethos to a new, professional style, based around a core of unmarried career nurses at the Hospital. The change was symbolised by the decision to affiliate the Hospital with the Victorian Trained Nurses Association, which connected the

Hospital to the wider nursing profession. However, both Miss Middleton and Miss Lewers stayed only a short time and the scant evidence suggests that they encountered some opposition from the old style nurses still at the Hospital. Miss Lewers resigned in 1906 when the committee refused to support her when she disciplined Nurse Lena Dwyer, one of the longest serving members of the staff, for insubordination and disobedience.[9]

Miss Lewers was succeeded as matron by Mrs Rose Backhouse, the last married matron of the Hospital. Unfortunately we know nothing about Mrs Backhouse's origins or career, except that she was either divorced, separated or widowed and that the committee allowed her young son to live at the Hospital with her. Mrs Backhouse was clearly not in the mould of the unmarried career nurses who were increasingly dominating the nursing profession, but her career again foundered after a conflict with Lena Dwyer, which led the committee to dismiss both of them.

It seems likely that the next matron, Miss M. Hooley, played a vital role in the professionalisation of nursing at the Warrnambool Hospital. She remained at the Hospital for eight years, the equal longest term of any matron in this period, and her frequent threats of resignation suggest that she encountered some opposition to her methods. However, the committee always supported her and when she finally left in 1914 she received a glowing testimonial.

The next matron, Miss Reeves, was another career nurse. She had been at the Hospital for only a year when she asked the committee for permission to enlist for overseas service and, although the committee was willing to hold her position open for her, she chose to resign in 1916. Her successor, Miss A.V. Anderson, was noted for her efficiency and professionalism, seeing the Hospital through the crisis of the 1919 influenza epidemic with a minimum of disruption. She was followed by Miss Warrender Davidson, who had been the Hospital's first trainee to pass the V.T.N.A. examinations in 1904, but we know little of her, or her successor, Miss Peacock.

Miss Lucy Paton, matron from 1924 to 1926, was another graduate of the Hospital's nurse training school. Thelma Hance, who trained during Miss Paton's term as matron, remembers her as very competent and dignified. Miss Paton's departure from the Hospital was very sudden. In her report dated 30 September 1926 she wrote, "I hereby make an application for an increase to £170 in my annual salary, as my responsibilities are daily increasing. I trust you will give favourable consideration to my request and thankyou in anticipation." Her trust was misplaced, her request was refused and she resigned.[10]

Miss Paton's successor, Miss Jessie McKenzie, stayed only a short time at the Hospital, with her brief tenure being dominated by a conflict with the secretary over the delineation of their duties. Miss McKenzie, who had had "wide experience as matron of different country hospitals throughout the State",[11] understandably objected to having to carry out the secretary's duties in his absence without recognition or remuneration.[12] Miss McKenzie was followed by Miss Griffiths, who held the post for eight years, and is remembered by nurses of the period as being very fair and helpful, always having the welfare of the nurses at heart. Miss Griffiths' successor, Miss Little, was another career nurse in the same mould, who had trained in Launceston before moving to Victoria in the early 1920s. She worked at Yarram, Wangaratta, the Queen Victoria Hospital, and in New Zealand, before being appointed matron of the Warrnambool Base Hospital in 1935. Miss Little saw the Hospital through the period of rapid expansion in the late 1930s, before being appointed matron of the Ballarat Base Hospital in 1939. She returned to Launceston in 1947, where she ran an electrolysis practice for many years, and died in 1988 at the age of eighty-nine.[13]

[1] Sister Thelma Hance (Mrs Thelma Surridge), "Nursing in Warrnambool in the Mid-1920s," unpublished address to the Warrnambool Hospital Past Trainees Association, 40th reunion, 26 March 1987 in WBHA.
[2] Matrons' Report Book, 6 January 1921.
[3] Matrons' Report Book, 1 September 1921.
[4] For example, Matron's Report Book, 30 April 1928.
[5] Reminiscences of Thelma Surridge, pp.19–20.
[6] Committee Minutes, March and April 1906, January 1908.
[7] *Standard*, 19 January 1937.
[8] Committee Minutes, 3 October 1906.
[9] Committee Minutes, March and April 1906.
[10] Matrons' Report Book, 30 September and 31 October 1926.
[11] *Standard*, 12 November 1926.
[12] Matrons' Report Book, April 1927.
[13] I am grateful to Mrs M. Jamieson née Marfell of Barwon Heads for this information on Miss Little.

Chapter 11

THE SECOND WORLD WAR

The Second World War was a critical period. During the late 1930s the Hospital had made the step from being a local hospital to a true regional base hospital, with the appropriate buildings, facilities, staff and financial base. However, the gains were still in a fragile and immature state and it was highly possible that some of them would be lost during the turmoil and disruption of the war years.

The Hospital's final annual report before the start of the war was one of the most satisfactory in its history. The committee reported that the new buildings and facilities erected over the previous decade were all in full use and functioning smoothly. The finances were in good shape despite a steep rise in the number of patients over the previous three years. The nursing staff had grown considerably to cope with the increased number of patients and the introduction in 1938 of a fifty hour week for nurses. The Hospital had twenty-two trained sisters and forty trainees—a far better ratio of trained staff to trainees than most hospitals had at the time. The committee acknowledged the high level of community support which had made the rapid progress of the previous few years possible.[1]

In total contrast to the enthusiasm which greeted the start of the First World War, the outbreak of war in September 1939 was met with grim resignation in Australia. To a very large extent society tried to maintain a "business as usual" approach and the full impact of war was not felt until Japan entered the War in December 1941. Within a few weeks of the declaration of war the Hospital's egg appeal went ahead as normal, with the *Standard* noting that "the fact that we are at war should not make any difference in the response to this appeal".[2] This attitude was maintained, with increasing difficulty, for the first two years of the War.

The most dramatic early impact of the War arose from the widespread belief that it would begin with extensive destruction of cities by vast fleets of bombers. Councillor N.K. Morris was the head of Warrnambool's air raid precautions and on the day of the outbreak of the war he advised the citizens that "We do not anticipate an air raid on Warrnambool within the next twenty-four hours", but he could give no assurances beyond that.[3] In October 1939 Councillor Morris attended a hospital committee meeting to explain air raid and evacuation procedures:

> He hoped for co-operation from the Hospital and if the necessity arose it would be practicable to evacuate the patients to some distant centre, maybe Hamilton would be the centre for the Hospital. It would be necessary that motor trucks and other vehicles, such as Nestlés lorries, be utilised for evacuation purposes . . . There was no experience to guide them in the matter of hospital evacuation and the removal of patients of a Base Hospital would involve a considerable problem . . . It would be advisable if someone attached to the Hospital attended the Air Raid Precautions instructional class to be held in Warrnambool shortly, and he thought that their Radiologist, Dr. Patrick, who had had experience in France, would be most suitable.[4]

After the initial flurry of concern over possible air raids and evacuation, the Hospital settled down to the more mundane problems of wartime. These can be summarised in the word that almost typifies the war years on the home front, "shortages". The Hospital faced shortages of staff, supplies and money, and the staff and the committee spent much of the war years attempting to overcome these problems.

There was an acute shortage of doctors throughout the War. Several of the honoraries, notably Doctors Berryman, Buzzard and Macknight, volunteered for service with the A.I.F., and this threw a great burden on the remaining doctors. For most of the War the Hospital functioned with just four senior medical staff. With the exception of Dr Patrick, the paid radiologist, the senior staff all gave their services to the Hospital on an honorary basis and relied on their private practices for their income. An increase in their hospital work almost inevitably involved a decrease in their incomes, but they responded to the crisis without complaint. Dr Horace Holmes had intended to retire in 1939, but he returned to work for the duration of the War when his successor, Dr Berryman, joined the A.I.F.

In contrast to the First World War, the Hospital was able to keep a resident doctor for most of the War. This was mainly because the controls of manpower in the Second World War enabled the authorities to ensure that all new medical graduates had at least a short hospital residency before joining the forces. In the early years of the War there were many short term residents, but in the later years, the Hospital obtained a resident doctor, Anthony Forshaw, who provided more continuity for the position. Dr Forshaw was married, which was most unusual for a resident in that period, and his wife had a baby in the Hospital in March 1944. The workload for the wartime residents must have been enormous, because of the absence of honoraries and because the number of patients continued to rise. In the early 1940s the average number of patients was over three times the average number when the first resident had been appointed.

The Hospital was acutely short of trained nurses throughout the war years. Until the last year of the War there was no shortage of trainee nurse applicants, but there were never enough sisters to train them properly and to maintain the services of the Hospital. The demand for nurses from the armed forces was very high and many trained nurses left to enlist, while others went to the city where similar shortages gave them excellent opportunities for promotion and experience. Throughout the war the *Standard* had stories such as this one from September 1941:

> ACUTE STAFFING POSITION AT HOSPITAL
>
> The acute staffing position at the Warrnambool Hospital was debated at the monthly meeting of the committee on Thursday night, following upon the announcement of the resignation of two of the sisters. The secretary said that efforts to secure locally trained staff to take up such positions had failed, and he had tried to secure nurses from Melbourne, Ballarat, Hamilton and other Western District centres without success, although offering high wages. They could get trainees, but they could get no one to train them, and the position was intensified by the fact that all the Hospital wards were full.[5]

One result of the shortage of trained nurses was that the Hospital began to employ married nurses for the first time since the old days of the "master and mistress". Many local women had trained as nurses and, as was universal at the time, left upon getting married. However, from 1941 married nurses were welcomed on the staff, with Sister J. Thompson (née Elliott) being among the first.

Up until this time all nurses had lived at the Hospital as a matter of course, in strictly regulated and disciplined conditions. The aims of this were to have the nurses close at hand and, more importantly, to give the nurses the security which single women were then regarded as needing—in effect the Hospital undertook the role of chaperone for its nurses. Unfortunately even the most tightly controlled conditions could not always protect the nurses from the realities of the world. This was tragically illustrated in late 1941 when a nurse was charged with murder following the death of her newborn baby in her bedroom.

Ruth Anderson, charge sister, c.1939–40

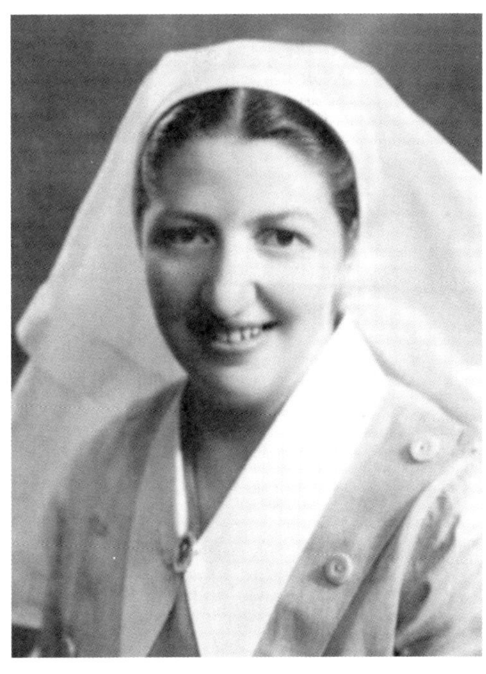

Throughout the War the Hospital found it hard to recruit the full complement of wardsmaids and housemaids, as the women who usually filled these positions were able to get better paid employment in food and munitions factories both locally and in Melbourne. One result of this was that wages for cleaners and domestics at the Hospital rose substantially, but to some extent their work was done by volunteers and the nurses.

The administration was also short-staffed during the war. The secretary and manager, John Plummer, joined the RAAF in June 1942 and his replacement, Mr W. Stoffel of Ararat, appears to have never actually taken up his position. As the Hospital also lacked an accountant at the time, the running of the Hospital devolved on a youthful Stewart Lindsay. Mr Lindsay was eventually appointed manager when Mr Plummer took up a position in Ballarat on leaving the air force, and he went on to a highly distinguished career as the Hospital's longest serving chief executive.

The War inevitably led to a squeeze on the Hospital's finances. There had been a rapid rise in the income and expenditure of the Hospital in the five years before the War and, as the number of patients continued to rise, the expenditure also continued to rise. However, in wartime conditions, the government grant only grew slowly, and in 1942 it actually fell. Similarly it became much harder to raise money locally as there were far more demands on people's charity for innumerable war-related causes such as the Red Cross, prisoners of war as well as the many government war loans. The problem was compounded for the Hospital because the Red Cross was not able to maintain its role with the auxiliary during the War, and this made it very difficult for the auxiliary to maintain the level of their

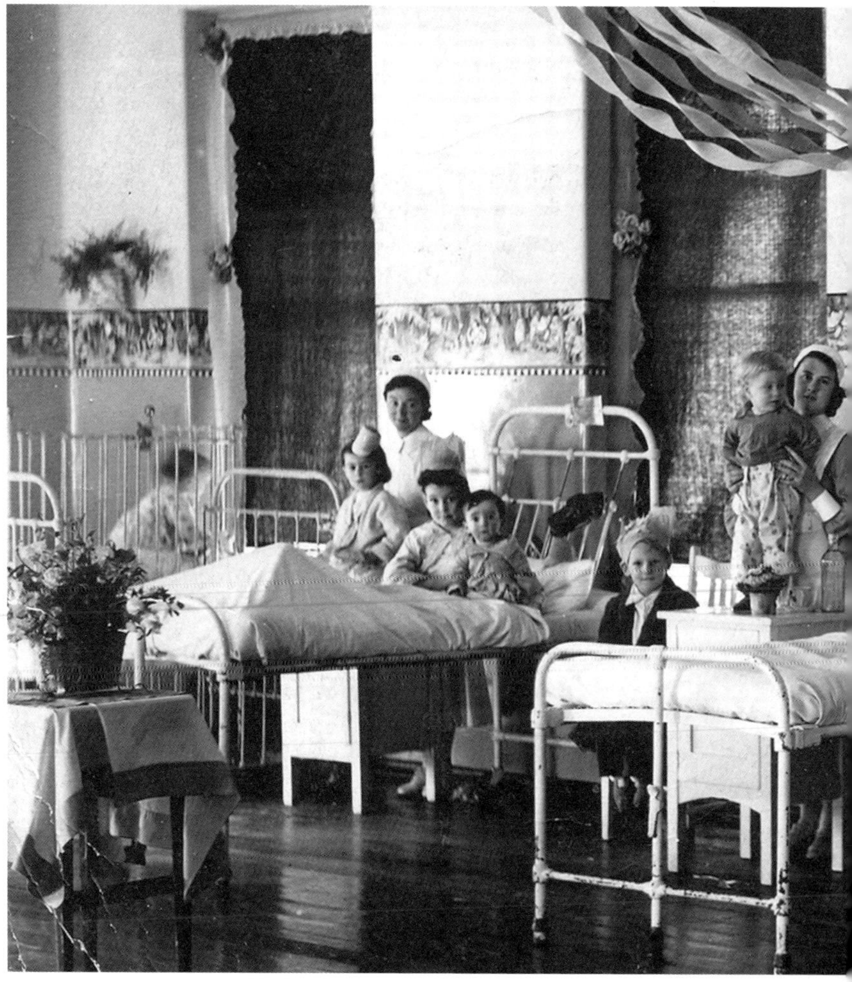

contributions to the Hospital. Mrs Pattison, the president of the auxiliary explained the situation in her annual report in July 1943:

> During the year we have had a change of name, the peace-time work of the Warrnambool branch of the Red Cross has been mainly hospital auxiliary, but now the Red Cross is working as was originally intended—the succour of sick and wounded in war time—we are not allowed to use the name Red Cross in any other sense, so we now work as a separate identity under the name of the Warrnambool Base Hospital Auxiliary . . . It has been a quiet but useful year of work for our sewing groups, curtailed, of course, by the rationing restrictions.[6]

One of the few hospital departments which did not suffer too severely from shortages during the War was the pharmacy. This was due to the foresight of the pharmacist, Jean Lineker, who had anticipated wartime supply problems and purchased large quantities of items most in demand. Consequently the Warrnambool Hospital was one of the very few country

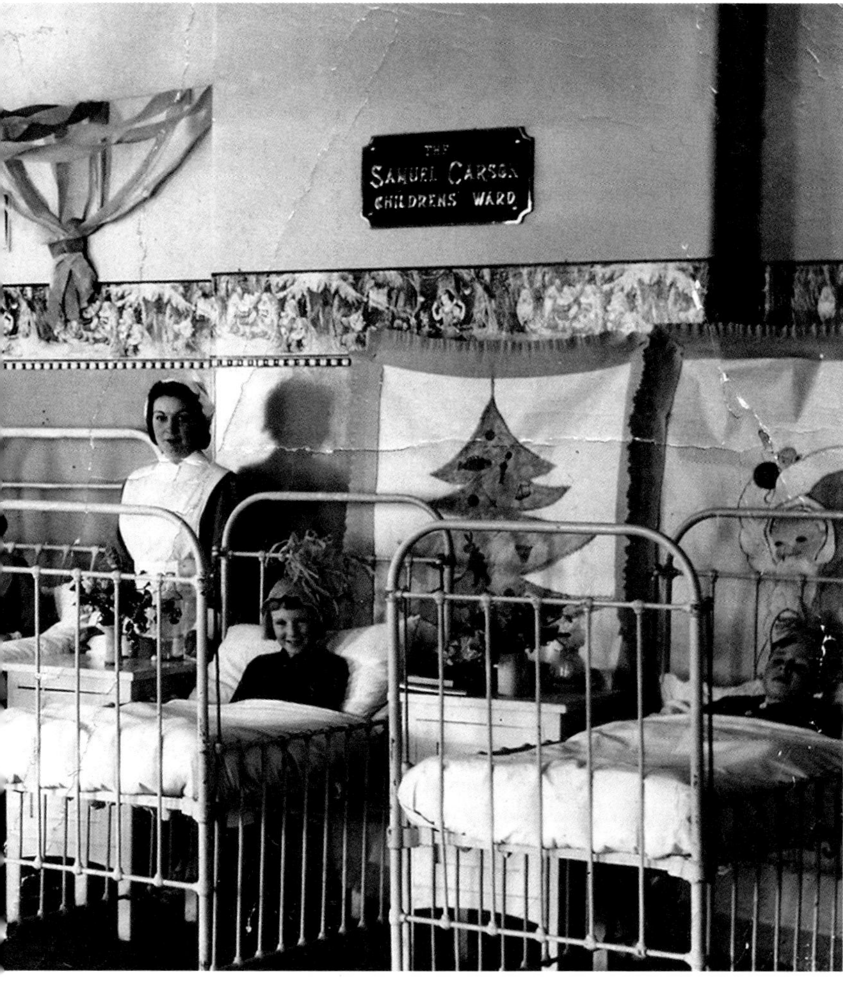

Children's ward, 1940

hospitals not to suffer from shortages of vital medicines during the war years.[7]

Fear of enemy attack was only an important factor in the Hospital's planning for the twelve months following the Japanese offensive in south-east Asia in December 1941. There was a renewed sense of urgency in the air raid precautions: the roof was covered with red crosses, the x-ray department was completely shrouded with fine mesh wire to decrease ray emissions, and large trenches for air raid shelters were dug in the lawns around the Hospital. The most difficult task was observing the strict blackout as the Hospital had over 700 windows of all shapes and sizes which had to be covered to prevent the slightest chink of light showing.[8] Stewart Lindsay recalls that the Hospital received confidential orders for full evacuation of patients and staff by train to central Victoria in the event of an enemy invasion.[9]

Fortunately air raids and invasion did not eventuate, but wartime conditions led to some different problems. The shortage of doctors, poor wartime diet, lack of quality controls especially with the milk supply, and parental absence and related factors contributed to a decline in the health of Warrnambool's children and a sharp rise in admissions to the children's and infectious diseases wards.[10] In 1943 Warrnambool experienced its first diphtheria epidemic for twenty years. Dr Holmes reported that early cases had not been treated and three patients had died. Altogether seventy-seven patients were admitted to the Hospital before the epidemic faded. This outbreak prompted a mass vaccination campaign—about 1450 children in Warrnambool were inoculated against diphtheria in late 1943.[11]

As the immediate threat to Australia receded from 1943, there was much effort throughout the country devoted to planning for post-war reconstruction. This was very much in evidence at the Hospital and in the last two years of the War it made several important innovations and planned many more. The pathological laboratory, which had been closed early in the war, was reopened in September 1943. Mr William Straede was appointed head of the department and he greatly expanded the range of its activities.[12] In June 1944 the Hospital established a blood bank. Previously blood had had to be obtained for each transfusion, normally from a relative of the patient, and the new blood bank gave the Hospital a permanent supply for the first time.[13]

The sharp increase in the number of children admitted during the War placed great pressure on the children's ward. The matron frequently commented on this in her monthly reports to the committee. For example, in August 1943 she stated that "The children's ward had been taxed to the utmost and the absence of suitable cots and observation wards had caused conditions which left much to be desired."[14] Consequently a new children's ward became a chief priority for post-war plans. Initially, in the spirit of extravagant optimism which characterised many plans for post-war reconstruction, the Hospital envisaged building a large free-standing children's block. However, reality forced these plans to be scaled down, so that the provision of a new children's ward became the target. Much of the fundraising in the latter years of the War was devoted to financing this ward.

Another project which had its genesis in the later years of the war was a "T.B. chalet" for sufferers from tuberculosis. In August 1944 the *Standard* reported:

> Some time ago the committee of the Warrnambool and District Base Hospital brought under the notice of Mr. H.S. Bailey, M.L.A., the great necessity for a T.B. chalet at the institution. It was pointed out that there was constantly as many as ten T.B. cases in the Hospital at the same time, and facilities were not available for dealing properly with such cases . . . Mr Bailey has advised "The Standard" that Mr. Macfarlane [the Minister for Public Health] has expressed sympathy towards the proposal.[15]

Mr Macfarlane visited Warrnambool soon after and Stewart Lindsay reported to him that in the previous two years there had been nineteen cases of tuberculosis in the Hospital, six of whom had died, and that the average length of stay of a TB patient was 121 days.[16] Mr Macfarlane promised assistance for a separate chalet for tuberculosis cases and, after the inevitable delays due to wartime shortages, the chalet was opened in 1946. Stewart Lindsay recalled that the Hospital contracted to buy the Hospital unit from the RAAF base at Cressy, "but on arrival to measure for transfer, it was half demolished, having been sold by another Government Department."[17] Eventually the Hospital was able to secure the officers' quarters from the base and these were cut up into moveable portions, transported to Warrnambool and placed on stumps prepared in the grounds in Ryot Street, close to the present main entrance. There were thirty-five beds which were immediately occupied, and a large waiting list soon developed.

The Hospital was also deeply involved in planning for future growth, inspired by a call by Mr McVilly, the Chief Inspector of Charities, that it should plan at least fifteen years in advance. After a children's ward, the most urgent need was seen to be extensions to the nurses' home, followed by a complete refurbishment of all the wards.[18]

While the Second World War had a substantial impact on the Hospital, much of its routine work continued without change throughout the War. The staff continued to care for patients presenting with a wide range of diseases, infections, and injuries. Naturally much of their work differed substantially from that of their metropolitan colleagues. A case which illustrates this was reported by Dr Littlewood in 1943:

> I was called to attend a boy about eight years of age suffering severe pain in the right side of the chest; he had a bad cough and expectoration which his parents told me he had since infancy. I diagnosed a bronchiectatic cavity with an attack of pleurisy. I ordered poultices which gave him relief. A few days later a pustule developed over the site of his pain; a day or two later his mother asked me to see him again as a hair seemed to be sticking out of the pustule. On visiting him I caught the so-called hair in a pair of forceps, and to my surprise I pulled out a complete head of

barley grass fully two and a half inches long, quite soft and flexible, coated with lymphy pus . . . Where did it come from?

On questioning the parents I found that the lad when about three years old had a violent attack of coughing, and seemed as if he would choke. This continued for at least a week, and ever since he had had a constant cough with profuse expectoration. After the removal of the grass head his symptoms cleared up completely.

My only explanation is that the grass head was pushed up the nose or by mouth entered the trachea through the larynx, passed into a bronchus, and eventually found its way to the pleura, and so through the chest wall.[19]

The late 1930s had seen a quickening of the pace of medical progress, particularly with the introduction of the sulpha drugs and blood transfusions. However, the range of diseases seen at the Hospital, and the prognosis for most of these diseases was little different from twenty or even forty years earlier. Diseases like polio, tuberculosis, rheumatic fever, osteomyelitis, diphtheria were widespread, and treatments for them were slow or ineffective. Massive infections were common and almost untreatable. The range of surgery was limited, not so much by surgical techniques as by primitive anaesthetics and the dangers of infection. Medicine was restricted to a small number of curative drugs—quinine, salvarsan, and the sulpha drugs—which were either applicable only to a few illnesses or else had severe side effects. Most other drugs only relieved symptoms or were purely placebos that would have looked more at home in a medieval book of folk remedies than in a modern hospital pharmacy. However, the Second World War saw extraordinarily rapid progress in medical science, with the result that both medicine and surgery were transformed during the 1940s. It is probably true to say that the 1940s saw greater medical progress than any decade in human history, with the possible exception of the 1860s.[20]

During the Second World War many members of the Hospital staff served in the medical services of the armed forces. The high standard of their training and wide experience at a major country hospital enabled them to make an important contribution to the war effort. The haphazard fortunes of war meant that their experiences varied from the dramatic to the mundane, from the tragic to the pedestrian.

The fate of the Australian nurses evacuated from Singapore in February 1942 was among the most horrific events of the war. Two former trainees of the Warrnambool Base Hospital, Wilma Oram and Mona Wilton, were among the nurses evacuated on the *Vyner Brooke*. Wilma Young (nee Oram) has told their story:

My name is Wilma Young née Oram. It was my privilege to train at the Warrnambool Base Hospital at the same time as Mona Wilton in the 1930s.

Mona was senior to me and we were on night duty together—she in the Women's ward and myself in the Children's ward—so we worked very closely together. We shared all our duties, including having to stoke the hot water boiler during the night!

I well remember the night we had five admissions and five deaths, and by the morning we were in a state of hysterical shock. Mona was a very efficient, happy nurse who was loved by all her patients, for whom she was very caring.

Some time after we finished our training, when our country was at war, Mona and I found ourselves together once again in the same unit (the 13th AGH) and we were sent to Singapore. Our first two weeks were spent becoming acclimatised: we gave lectures to our orderlies and enjoyed the social life. Mona and I shared all our letters from home and we always went on leave together, so we literally shared our lives throughout our time together.

From Singapore Mona and I, along with some other nurses, were sent to Johore Bahru on the Malaysian peninsula, where we joined the 2/4th CCS [casualty clearing station]. Later we became a fully functioning General Hospital when the CCS moved out. The Hospital was a mental hospital, which had to be adapted to our use, and was always very primitive.

Mona carried out all her duties with great care and always with her patients' well-being at the forefront of her endeavours. Her good humour and her wit endeared her to all who knew her. She was well loved by all who had dealings with her and when word came that we were to evacuate Singapore to be sent home, her patients were devastated. Mona too was devastated, for her one desire was to stay to give succour to her patients, but it was not to be.

We nurses were ordered to board a ship called the SS *Vyner Brooke* to leave Singapore amidst heavy fighting and air raids. After a day and a half at sea, our ship was bombed and sunk in the Bangka Strait.

Mona and I were below deck when this happened, and one of our nursing colleagues was wounded. Mona helped to carry her up on to the upper deck, where her wound was dressed and she was placed in one of the life-boats. Tragically, however, this nurse was later to become one of the victims of a Japanese massacre—being shot alongside twenty-one of her nursing colleagues on a beach on Bangka Island. Vivian Bullwinkel was the only nurse to survive this massacre.

Mona and I escaped from the rapidly sinking ship into a life-boat, but as the life-boat was sinking and the *Vyner Brooke* was beginning to tip over on top of us, we jumped out of the boat and tried to get away from the ship. As neither of us could swim, this was a very difficult situation. Eventually, the ship did tip over on top of us, and Mona was drowned. Somehow, I managed to struggle out.

Mona was cheerful and full of hope right to the end.

Farewell my well-beloved friend, with whom I shared so much, and who had so much to give.[21]

Wilma Oram was taken prisoner by the Japanese and survived three and a half years of extraordinary brutality and privations.

Doris Swinton had a very different war experience. A member of one of Warrnambool's leading retailing families, she was born in 1904 and educated at Warrnambool Primary School and Warrnambool High School before training as a nurse at the Royal Melbourne Hospital. In 1931 she returned to Warrnambool to run Alveston Private Hospital. After three years she went to England where she worked at many of the leading hospitals in London. When war threatened in 1939 she joined the Queen Alexandra's Imperial Military Nursing Service and spent her wartime nursing service with the British Army. Doris was with the British Expeditionary Force in France and had some harrowing experiences during the retreat to the Channel and the evacuation to England.

Doris's next posting was to the Middle East where she nursed in Egypt, the Sudan and Palestine, often in very primitive conditions. After D Day she was with the British Army during the liberation of France, Belgium and Holland and the invasion of Germany. During the campaign in Europe she was in charge of a casualty clearing station and was frequently under shellfire. It was during this time that Matron Swinton was twice mentioned in despatches, and in March 1945 she received an M.B.E. (military division) for her outstanding wartime service. She was one of the most highly decorated Australian nurses in the Second World War. She returned to Australia to great acclaim in November 1946 and in 1948 she became Matron of the Warrnambool Base Hospital, becoming one of the most distinguished figures in the Hospital's history.[22]

[1] *Standard*, 17 August 1939.
[2] *Standard*, 13 September 1939.
[3] *Standard*, 5 September 1939.
[4] *Standard*, 13 October 1939.
[5] *Standard*, 13 September 1941.
[6] *Standard*, 20 July 1943.
[7] *Standard*, 30 April 1944.
[8] *Standard*, 30 December 1941.
[9] Notes by Stewart Lindsay, August 1997.
[10] The same factors were at work throughout Australia. The Royal Children's Hospital in Melbourne experienced a sharp rise in admissions of children with malnutrition and an upsurge in the numbers with infectious diseases such as diphtheria and typhoid which had been declining in the years before the war.
[11] *Standard*, 2 February 1944.
[12] *Standard*, 23 September 1944.
[13] *Standard*, 24 June 1944. The first eleven regular donors were Miss E. Duggan and Messrs Arthur Haberfield, Don Martin, Arthur Savage, R.A. Smith, S.G. Tinker, Alan Greed, C.G.W. Hunt, C.P. McKenna, W.T.C. Straede and E. Trotter.
[14] *Standard*, 23 August 1943.
[15] *Standard*, 4 August 1944.
[16] *Standard*, 15 August 1944.
[17] Notes by Stewart Lindsay, August 1997.
[18] *Standard*, 19 July 1944.
[19] F.E. Littlewood, "A Grass Seed in the Lung," *Medical Journal of Australia*, 5 June 1943, p.524.
[20] In the 1860s, Pasteur established that germs were responsible for disease and infection, and Lister applied this knowledge to develop antiseptic surgery.
[21] Wilma Young, "Tribute to Mona Wilton", unpublished mss 1998.
[22] Maureen Johnstone, "A Character Profile of a Nurse who has made a Significant Contribution to Nursing — Doris Anne Swinton (Matron Swinton)", unpublished mss. 1993; *Standard*, 5 July 1944.

Chapter 12

THE MEDICAL REVOLUTION

On 10 May 1944, the following report appeared in the *Standard*:

> At a meeting of the board of management of the Warrnambool and District Base Hospital on Thursday night, the secretary, Mr S.A. Lindsay, reported that during the week a case in the public section of the institution had been successfully treated with the wonder drug penicillin. Stocks of the drug were extremely limited and were only released under the control of penicillin order prescribed under the National Security Regulations. Mr Lindsay said that eight diseases only were listed, for which application could be made, and a disease must be verified by bacteriological examination.

Australia was the first country in the world to have supplies of penicillin available for civilian use and, as this only occurred in April 1944, it indicates that the Warrnambool Hospital was among the earliest hospitals in the world to use penicillin on a civilian.

The nurses of the time recall that the advent of penicillin involved much extra work for them:

> It took two to make it up and it had to be kept in the fridge and the only fridge was down in the kitchen and you gave the penicillin every three hours. And when it was time to give it, you rolled down your sleeves, you put on your cuffs, you went to the kitchen, you got the key, you unlocked the fridge, you got the penicillin, you locked the fridge, you took the key back to the housekeeper, back to the ward and you took your cuffs off and rolled your sleeves up. The penicillin was given under quite a lot of supervision . . . and after you gave the injection you rolled down your sleeves and put your cuffs on, went back to the kitchen and went through all that rigmarole in reverse and by the time you got back to the ward it was time to start again. There were two to give it because one had to scrub and remain sterile and the other one had to get the patient ready.
>
> All the making up of the penicillin was initially done under Miss Lineker's supervision until we were really competent and able to go ahead with it because it was so precious and so expensive.[1]

The introduction of penicillin was the greatest single step in the revolution which transformed medicine in the 1940s and 1950s. The development of antibiotics and the spread of immunisation changed long-established patterns of disease, with many diseases disappearing or becoming readily curable. Diseases like osteomyelitis, tuberculosis, poliomyelitis, bronchiectasis, diphtheria, and nephritis, which filled the wards of hospitals before the Second World War, had become very rare by 1960. Antibiotics and improvements in anaesthetic techniques greatly extended the potentialities of surgery and enabled surgeons to undertake a far wider range of operations. The most obvious example is the development of cardiac surgery, but progress was seen across the whole range of surgery from the correction of many previously fatal congenital abnormalities to trauma surgery.

The revolution in medicine transformed the work of the Hospital. In 1943 the board of management adopted a master plan for the development of the Hospital, which provided for a total of 365 beds. Given the patterns of disease at the time and projections for population growth, this appeared to be a sensible plan. However, the rapid changes in medicine greatly reduced both the number of hospital admissions relative to the population and the average length of stay in hospital. At the opening of the main ward block in 1963, the chairman of the Hospital and Charities Commission, Dr J. Lindell, stated that progress in medical science had reduced the number of hospital beds needed by about half.[2] As a result, the number of beds provided at the Warrnambool Base Hospital reached a peak of about 180 in 1970 and has been steadily declining since then. The average length of stay was twenty-two days in 1943, twelve days in 1954 and five days in 1972.

Until the 1940s a high proportion of patients were long term. For many chronic conditions such as osteomyelitis and tuberculosis of the bones and joints, the only treatment was immobility and rest and patients frequently spent years in hospital. In addition the Hospital still had a large number of geriatric patients, as there was nowhere else in the district to care for the large number of old people who could neither be cared for at home nor afford private hospital care.

By the 1970s, many chronic illnesses had been eliminated. Many other chronic patients were able to be cared for at home, thanks to the development of such services as visiting nurses and Meals on Wheels. The inappropriate use of acute hospital beds for long term geriatric patients was gradually reduced when the Hospital took over the old "Alveston" and "Corio" private hospitals and by the development of Lyndoch into a major geriatric centre.

Essie Smith of Naringal had two lengthy periods in the Hospital in the late 1940s and early 1950s and her experiences give a good picture of the work of the Hospital in those years.

> I had always been a healthy person. Then on 18 April 1945 I went into a diabetic coma at Dr Buzzard's place, in his surgery. My husband took me to hospital and I was admitted to ward two, the female ward. It was a very long ward with ten or twenty beds down either side.
>
> I don't remember much for about three days because I was . . . in a very deep coma for three days. I remember the nurses coming in. I didn't know then that I was diabetic, but I wondered why every now and then they

were putting needles in my arm. They woke me up at terrible hours of the morning and I can remember one nurse giving me an apple at two o'clock in the morning, and that I had to eat every piece of it, and I was so weak that I couldn't.

I came out of the coma and I had a little screen around me. I can remember Dr Buzzard well . . . He looked over the top of the screen and he said to me, "Well, St Peter didn't get you."

A few days after I lost my eyesight. I can remember that they took me from my ward down to a dark room in Marcus Saltau House and put a cover over my eyes. I can still remember hearing the visitors to the other patients saying, "Oh that poor dear over there, she's gone blind." In about a week my eyesight came back.

The nurses were wonderful and I can still remember their names. They were wonderful because they were very attentive and they had a very strict Matron . . .

I was pregnant with my first child. I was in the Hospital six weeks and two days before I was to come home I lost my baby.

From then on I had many trips to hospital, because in those days they didn't know a lot about diabetes. I was on insulin—these were the needles they were poking in my arm at all hours of the night and day . . .

In 1951 I was back in hospital with what they suspected was a "spot on the lung" . . . I had been so sick in those years my resistance had got low and I was rather skinny. They said I would be in hospital only for a short time, but because of complication I was in there for seventeen months continuously, in the building that is now the Laurel Club down in Banyan Street—the old chalet . . .

[The Tuberculosis Clinic was run by] Dr Williams, a lady doctor who used to come from Melbourne. They would take us to this dark room and we were all lined up and waiting. Some patients were seriously ill but I never was. The food they gave for the lung complaint they could not give me because of the diabetes, so they had to put me on a very special diet.

When we left the Hospital we would go back every fortnight to have air put in our lungs and we would meet up with all the patients we had met there and have a great old yarn . . . To put the air in your lungs, they came at me with a needle and go right through into your lung—it was no fun and it was painful. That happened once a fortnight until the doctor said I didn't need it anymore.

I was a dressmaker and I used to make my daughter's clothes by hand in the Hospital, and then I was allowed to bring my machine in . . . Sister Taylor, who was in charge of the chalet at the time, made her wedding dress on my machine.

After the seventeen months I came home and I was slicing some beans and got a pain and I thought "Oh, no" and I went back to the Hospital and they put me back in the chalet for another five months. It took two years of my life.

I have a lot to thank the Hospital for and the girls there.

While there were many patients like Essie Smith with long term chronic illnesses, another group of long term patients were not really sick at all. In

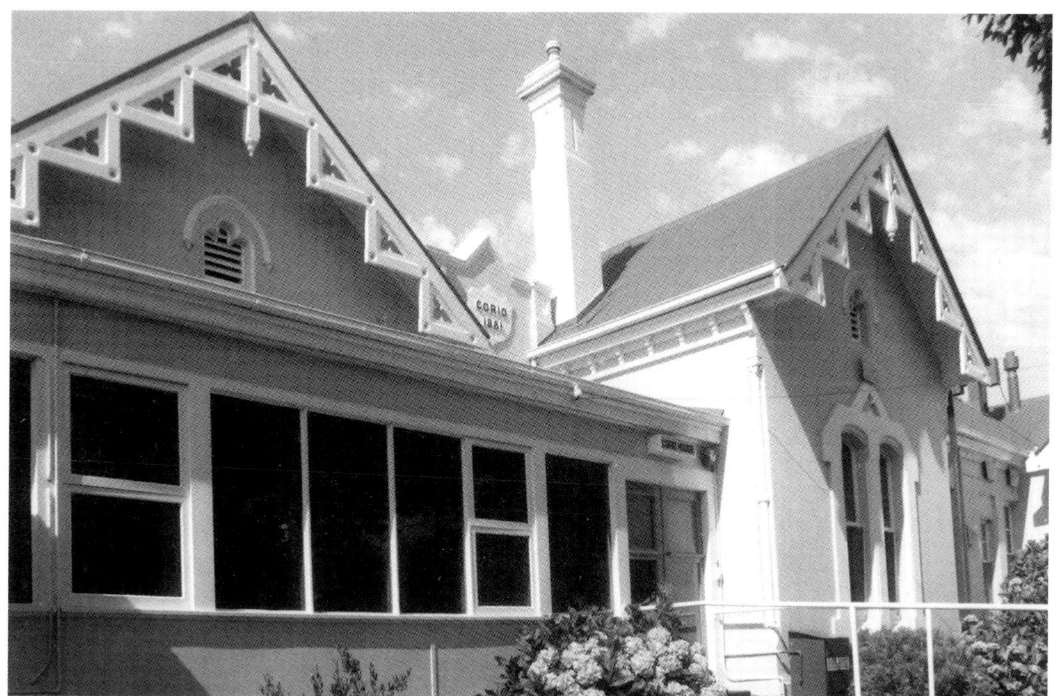

Corio House aged care facility

October 1956, Matron Swinton reported to the board of management that "The general wards are inundated with the chronically ill and senile patients, thus making the nursing difficult and rather uninteresting for the student nurses."[3] Several months later she noted that the adult wards were "being constantly filled with elderly patients mostly in a rather advanced state of helplessness."[4] The proper care of elderly people was a constant preoccupation of the Warrnambool community in the 1950s. The Hospital had originally been founded primarily as a benevolent home for the aged poor and, although its role as an acute hospital expanded continually, it proved very difficult to develop more appropriate accommodation for the elderly.

One consequence of having large numbers of patients who were in the Hospital because they were old and poor was that it was sometimes difficult to maintain the decorum expected in a hospital. A considerable number of these patients were alcoholics and staff members were frequently forced to cope with people suffering from *delirium tremens*. The Hospital had a continual problem with patients smuggling alcohol in. As late as 1966 the *Standard* reported:

> The Transport Regulation Board has warned Warrnambool taxi-drivers following complaints that taxis have been taking liquor to Warrnambool Hospital patients.
>
> It has been alleged that some taxi-drivers have been taking dozens of bottles to patients, particularly in male ward 7 on the medical floor. . . .
>
> The liquor allegedly brought by taxis had been delivered to patients

> without the knowledge of the sister-in-charge. It is believed that at least once, almost all patients in a ward were affected by liquor.[5]

Although the Hospital realised that there was a need for more appropriate accommodation for geriatric patients, it took many years before the problem was fully resolved. The first step came in the early 1950s when the Hospital took over responsibility for Alveston and Corio. These facilities had been functioning as private hospitals for many years, but under the Hospital's management they were adapted to cater exclusively for long term geriatric patients. The Hospital took over Alveston in August 1951 and fifteen months later the *Standard* described the institution:

> Every room has been repainted, floors have been resanded and lino laid down, and an electric bell system operates day and night from each patient's bed to the staff quarters. In addition to the front porch, a solarium at the back ensures that patients who can walk are not confined to their rooms even on the wettest days, as they can sit in comfortable armchairs and talk, smoke or read just as long as they desire.
>
> The grounds at the rear are laid out and planted with vegetables, which help considerably to keep down costs, and fresh eggs for the patients are gathered daily from the fowls in the newly-built fowlyard.
>
> A staff of 17 nurses and assistant nurses cares for the needs of the patients under the direction of Matron E. Smith . . . The capacity of the Home is 30 patients, and the great need for such an institution is demonstrated by the fact that there is always a waiting list of other old people desiring admission.
>
> The average age of the 30 inmates at present at Alveston is 78 years, the oldest being 93, another is 90, and several are in the late 80s. And—a most striking fact—every one of the present inmates comes from within a radius of 28 miles of Warrnambool.[6]

The Hospital took over the management of Corio in 1954, two years after the establishment of Lyndoch. Although it still took many years before the Warrnambool district had sufficient accommodation for elderly people, these events marked at least the beginnings of a solution. However, it is significant that the Hospital did not see the answer to the care of elderly people being a simple matter of providing sufficient beds. There was also an awareness of the value of aiding those who wanted to live in their own homes. As early as 1947 the Hospital employed a visiting nurse to provide home care primarily for elderly patients. Anticipating more recent trends, Dr Buzzard saw the visiting nurse service as helping to cut down the length of hospitalisation.[7]

Another important innovation which helped more elderly people stay in their own homes was the introduction of the Meals on Wheels service in the 1960s. This was a joint initiative of the Hospital and the Rotary Club, with the first meals being delivered in March 1965. By 1967 nearly 8000 meals were distributed annually by volunteer drivers, and in the years since the number has continued to grow, providing an invaluable service to the town's elderly citizens.

One of the most important changes at the Hospital in the years after the Second World War was the development of more humane attitudes toward patients. The origins of the Hospital as a benevolent institution for the sick poor had inevitably bred a paternalistic attitude toward the patients. The attitude appeared to be that recipients of charity should accept the strict regimentation, plain food and lack of privacy without complaint. These attitudes persisted even after the decline of the old benevolent functions. One important reason for this was the strong tendency of the medical profession in the 1930s and 1940s to see patients as "cases" rather than people. Many patients of the era recall hearing their doctor refer to them as "the leg in ward two" or "the appendix in ward three" rather than by their names.

As with most other hospitals of the time, the Warrnambool Hospital enforced strict rules on visiting, with very limited visiting being allowed even for very young children. Even in the mid-1940s the tendency was to restrict visiting further.[8] In the maternity ward, babies were kept separate from their mothers throughout the lengthy hospital stay which was then the norm after childbirth. The large open public wards had up to twenty beds and offered no privacy to patients.

The trend towards a more humane and personal approach to patients began in the 1950s. The first sign of this came in March 1954 when Mr Percy Parker, a committee of management member, raised the possibility of "installing movable partitions to provide more privacy for patients in the public section of the Hospital".[9] He noted that the beds in the public wards were very close together with very little privacy and successfully moved that light movable screens should be provided.

The following year the first step toward moderating the austere and rigid conditions of the maternity ward came when the Hospital provided two special cots so that some mothers could have their babies near their beds. This was extended in the early 1960s so that more babies could "room-in" with their mothers. However, it was not until the 1970s that the Hospital began to abandon the old "production line" approach to childbirth and gave mothers more say in the birthing process.

The area where restricted visiting caused most distress and damage was in the children's ward. In the 1930s and 1940s doctors and nurses had sought to limit visiting to children in hospital on the grounds that visitors could introduce infectious diseases and that visits upset the children. However, the decline in most infectious diseases reduced the impact of the first argument, and both research and experience in the 1940s and 1950s showed that restricted visiting was psychologically damaging for many children.[10] Consequently, visiting hours in the children's ward at the Warrnambool Hospital were gradually liberalised during the 1950s and in July 1960 the Hospital adopted open visiting for children. Later in the 1960s the Hospital began to make provision for mothers to stay with sick children who were fretting. In another move to make the experience less terrifying for children, the Hospital began to give children colouring books on admission and produced a booklet, "Jill and Johnny go to Hospital", to give children some idea of what to expect.

Although the general trend throughout this period was to liberalise visiting, the Hospital began for the first time to try to restrict the propensity of visitors to smoke in the wards. In August 1955 the *Standard* reported that "Smoking to excess by some visitors in hospital wards has caused distress to patients, particularly those with chest ailments, and the Board of Management will erect notices indicating that visitors must not smoke while visiting patients in wards."[11] However, the notices seem to have had little effect. In 1968 the board of management reiterated its policy of requesting visitors not to smoke, but smoking was not banned altogether except in the children's ward.

Even without consideration of improvements in medical treatment, the conditions for patients improved greatly in the years 1945–72. The large old wards were replaced with modern smaller wards which gave patients much greater comfort and privacy, as well as being more convenient for the staff. New facilities such as the casualty department, operating theatres and the intensive care unit, as well as a great expansion in the

Theatre staff. Sr Gillian Reich, nurses Gaye Murrihy and Marianne Astbury— 26 April 1962

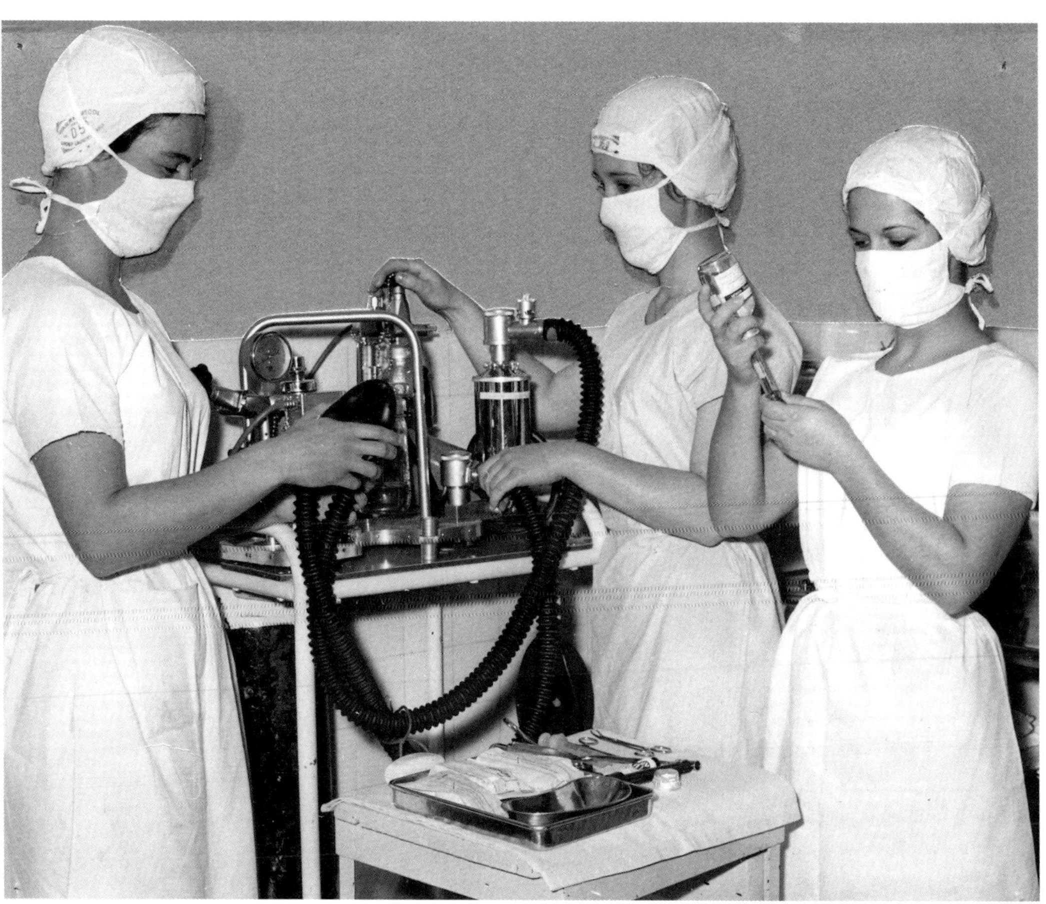

ancillary services offered by the Hospital, greatly increased the standard of patient care. These developments were accompanied by the Hospital's deliberate policy of becoming more humane in its treatment of patients.

The importance placed on the need to become more patient oriented is indicated by the frequency with which the need to remain focussed on patients as individuals was the main theme of the nursing graduation ceremonies. For example, in 1966, Mr Kel Gardiner, the Hospital's senior surgeon, reiterated to the graduates that the patient had to be the "focal point of all nursing"[12] and two years later, the matron, June Stewart, emphasised that "nurses should retain their humane ability as priority over their technical skills".[13]

[1] Interview with Thelma Surridge, June Stewart, Marion Trigg née Uebergang, Dorothy Crothers née Lee, Alison Stonehouse née McKenzie, Margaret Hudson née Donahue, Verna Whiteside née Pollack, Betty Taylor née Baulch, Doris Johnson née Baxter, Irene Bruce né9e Minogue, by Penny Forth, 5 August 1997.
[2] *Standard*, 18 November 1963.
[3] Board of Management Minutes, October 1956, p.37.
[4] Board of Management Minutes, January 1957, p.57.
[5] *Standard*, 1 March 1966.
[6] *Standard*, 8 November 1952.
[7] Committee of Management Minutes, October 1948, p.87.
[8] *Standard*, 29 March and 30 November 1946.
[9] *Standard*, 26 March 1954.
[10] Marion Ievers, Kate Campbell and Mona Blanch, "Unrestricted Visiting in a Children's Ward: eight years' experience," *Lancet*, 5 Nov. 1955, pp.971–73.
[11] *Standard*, 27 August 1955.
[12] *Standard*, 11 November 1966.
[13] *Standard*, 8 November 1968.

Chapter 13

THE HOSPITAL REBUILT 1945–1972

The transformation of the Warrnambool Base Hospital into a modern hospital began in the late 1930s with the construction of Marcus Saltau House. However, at the end of the Second World War, the physical appearance of the Hospital still had more in common with the old benevolent hospital of the nineteenth century than the modern base hospital of today. The period 1945 to 1972 saw the complete transformation of the Hospital, with the demolition of most of the old Hospital and the construction of many major new buildings. This phase of almost constant building projects took place during the lengthy term of Mr Stewart Lindsay, who stands out as the most influential administrator in the history of the Hospital, as secretary/manager.

Stewart Lindsay joined the Hospital staff as an administrative officer in the late 1940s. Soon after, the manager, Mr Plummer, joined the RAAF and his appointed replacement, Mr W. Stoffel, did not take up the position. Consequently Stewart Lindsay was effectively chief executive from soon after his arrival at the Hospital and, as the Hospital's accountant and the

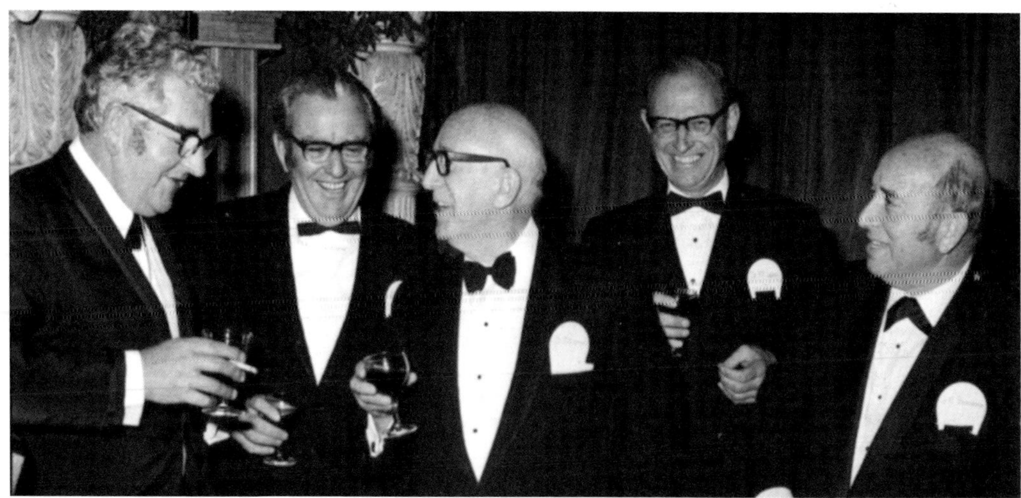

Official farewell for Stewart Lindsay, Town Hall, June 1972. V.G.C. Balmer, senior vice president; Geoff Bennett, junior vice president; Stewart Lindsay; Dr R.R. Sobey, president of the board of management and chairman of the function; Councillor H.I. Stephenson, mayor of the City of Warrnambool.

deputy manager were also in the armed forces, he was almost completely responsible for the whole administration. When Mr Plummer chose to take the manager's position at the Ballarat Hospital in December 1944, rather than return to Warrnambool, Stewart Lindsay was formally appointed manager, serving until his retirement in 1972.

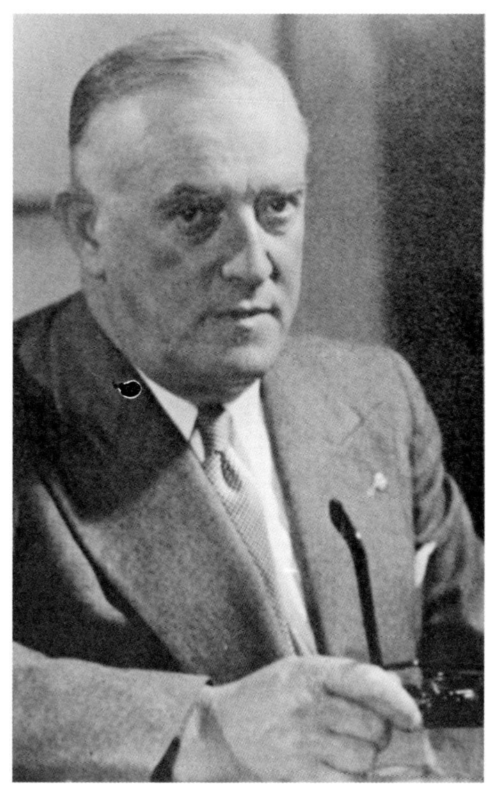

Rupert Philpott, member of board of management for 30 years, president 1944–45

Stewart Lindsay began work at the Hospital soon after the conclusion of Marcus Saltau's lengthy term as president. Where Marcus Saltau, as president, had been the driving force of the Hospital during the first phases of its modernisation, it was Stewart Lindsay, as manager, who was the driving force behind the rebuilding of the Hospital in the post-war years. The fact that Warrnambool had an outstanding and long-serving administrator in these years meant that the long term trend in Victorian hospitals for power to pass from elected boards to paid administrators could be seen here much earlier than in many other hospitals.

This trend was enhanced by the decision of the committee of management after the retirement of Marcus Saltau that there should be no more long term presidents. Consequently, since that time no president has held office for more than four years, and this has prevented any president developing the sort of dominant position that Marcus Saltau enjoyed.

The fundamental make-up of the committee of management remained largely unchanged in the decades after the end of the Second World War. With one exception, the committee was composed entirely of men, normally the leading businessmen of the town, with one or two doctors to present the views of the honorary medical staff.

The one woman to serve on the Hospital committee in this period was Mrs Helena Marfell. A leading figure in many community organisations, she was state president of the Country Women's Association from 1942 to 1945 and the first woman to stand for the federal seat of Wannon.[1] She became a member of the Hospital committee in 1945, in the first contested election for the committee since 1907.[2] It is perhaps significant that she had to win her place in an election rather than be offered a place when a vacancy occurred, which was the traditional way of joining the committee. She and her husband left Warrnambool in 1952 and, on her resignation from the committee, Mr J. McD. Taylor said he "thought it had been good for the committee to have a lady member, as her opinions had a freshness which was unusual but helpful."[3]

Children's ward exterior, pre-1962

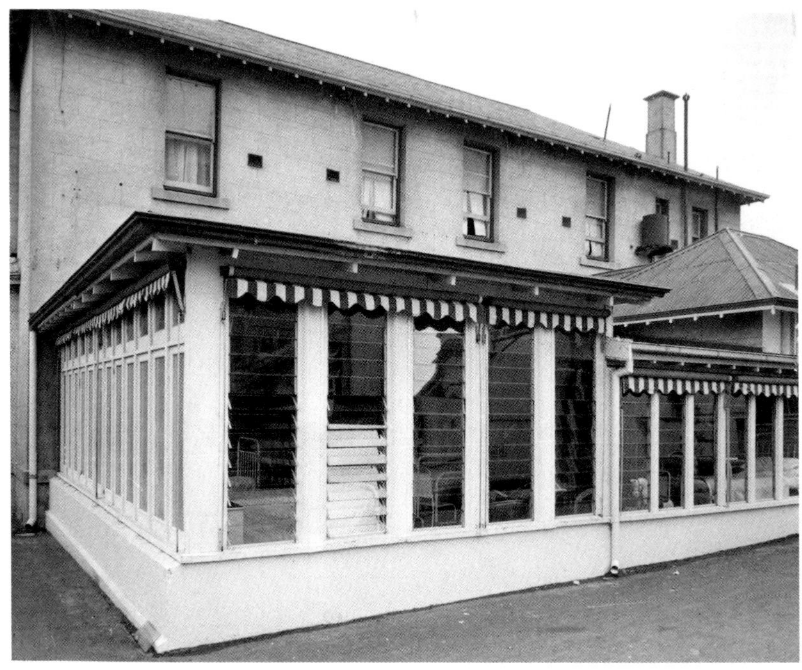

There has never been a period more conducive to long term planning than the last years of the Second World War. Throughout Australia, governments, businesses and institutions of all types threw themselves into planning for peacetime.[4] At the Warrnambool Hospital, planning began soon after Stewart Lindsay became acting manager. By September 1944 the *Standard* was able to report on the "complete long range plan to rebuild obsolete public sections of the Warrnambool and District Base Hospital". A leading hospital architect, Mr Robert Demaine, presented plans to the committee "for the suggested future development of the Hospital as a modern centre of health". The essential features of the "master plan" were:

> The proposed new block to house the children's ward will rise four floors above one of the solid single storey central sections of the existing hospital building. The first two floors will be the children's wards, the third and fourth will ultimately house the operating suite and a section of the men's ward . . .
>
> The building of the new children's ward will necessitate the demolition of portion of the nurses' quarters in the main hospital building, and will also mean an increase in the staff to cope with the extra children's ward bed accommodation. So simultaneously with the building of the children's section the board of management plans extension of the nurses' home, the present accommodation of which is inadequate housing only 40 of the nursing staff of 66.
>
> The ultimate development plan for the whole of the public section of the Hospital envisages the main block, extending from the new children's section due east toward Ryot Street. The ground floor is to house the administration, X-ray, dispensary and outpatients' services. The first and

second floors womens' wards and the third and fourth floors male wards. This scheme may take several years of gradual work, but it will be done to a concise plan that will combine an attractiveness of architecture with economy and utility.[5]

Before the development of the master plan the Hospital committee favoured the construction of a new children's ward as the most urgent building project. The need for this was very apparent as the original ward had been designed for seventeen beds, but by the early 1940s there were often over thirty children in the Hospital. The Hospital actually began a campaign to raise £5000 to finance the new ward even before the master plan was completed. This campaign was organised by Stewart Lindsay and Frank Ford and received widespread community support, with a flurry of "ugly men" competitions, market days, picnic race meetings and the like throughout 1943 and early 1944. The appeal greatly exceeded the target and by the end of March 1944 it had raised £11,800, an extraordinary achievement in wartime.[6]

While the War did not inhibit fundraising, it made building impossible as building permits, materials and labour were all unobtainable. Most of the money raised for the children's ward was set aside and, as it turned out, it remained set aside for many years. As the master plan developed, provision for the children's ward was to be in a multi-storeyed ward block, and there was no chance of constructing this in the 1940s.[7] The difficulties of building

Children's ward interior, pre-1962

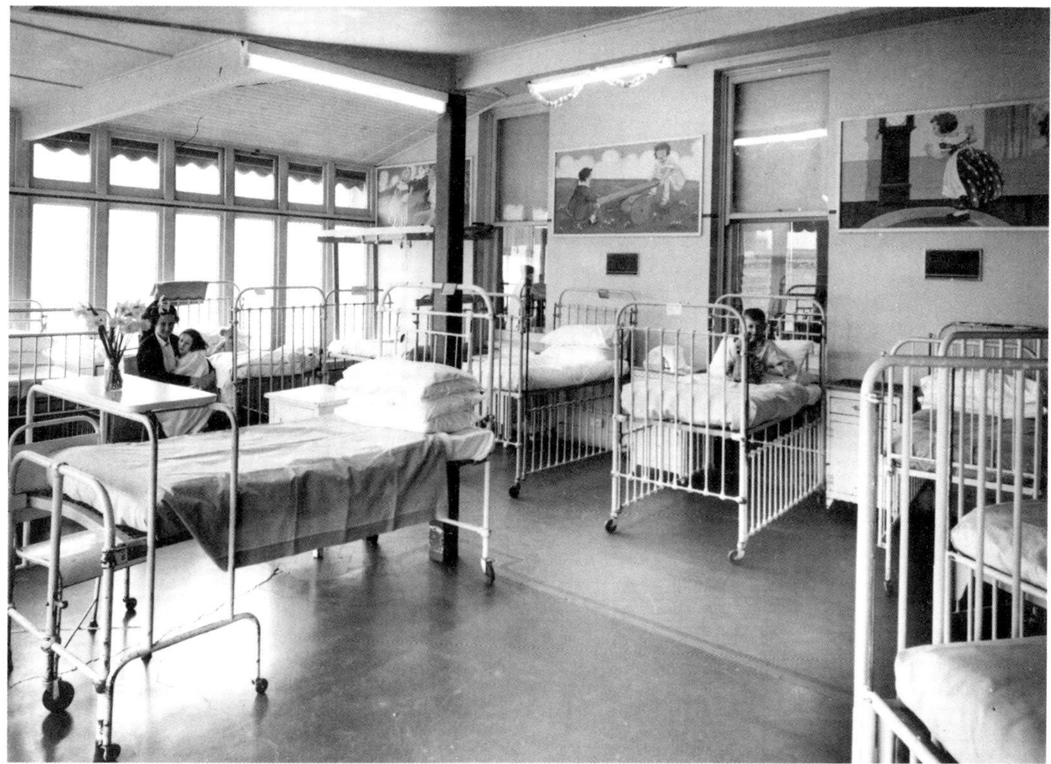

in the immediate post-war period, and a critical shortage of both nurses and nursing accommodation, made the construction of a new nurses' home seem a more urgent need than the children's ward. The committee of management believed that the Hospital would be able to attract more nurses if it was able to offer better accommodation for them. If the main ward block was constructed first, the Hospital would not have enough nurses to staff it.

Even after the Hospital made the decision to build a new nurses' home as the first stage of rebuilding the Hospital, it faced a lengthy delay before it was possible to begin work. In the post-war era there was enormous pent-up demand throughout Australia for new hospital buildings, and State and Federal Governments were not able to finance all of them, even if the labour and materials had been available. In spite of continuous lobbying, the Warrnambool Hospital did not receive a permit to begin work on the nurses' home until October 1948. Even after the permit had been granted, the Hospital faced continual delays with the project due to shortages, particularly of cement and money. The first of these was overcome by importing cement from Japan (still highly controversial soon after the War), and the financial shortfall was dealt with by means of a "community loan" whereby local people provided money for the Hospital, to be repaid when the Government came good on its promises.[8]

In October 1949 the Hospital committee accepted the tender of leading Warrnambool builder, Mr E.S. Harris, who was to carry out much of the construction work for the rebuilding of the Hospital. However, despite his best efforts, the new nurses' home was not completed until 1953. The *Standard* described the completed building:

> It contains 75 single bedrooms, four sitting rooms, two visiting rooms, lecture room, demonstration room, linen room, pantries, box rooms and general utilities.
>
> Consideration has been given to the use of colours in an attempt to obtain maximum warmth in winter and coolness in summer.
>
> An important part of the home is the training school, where nurses will be taught hospital routine preparing them for the responsibilities of ward duty and for qualification as trained nurses. . . .
>
> The new building is one which everyone connected with its planning may well be proud. It is worthy of the rapidly growing city and there is nothing shabby or shoddy to be found in the whole set up [except perhaps the roof which leaked for years!].[9]

The only other major works which were completed while the nurses' home was being built were the TB Chalet (discussed in chapter twelve) and the infectious diseases ward which was completed in 1947. Both these developments were anachronistic as progress in medical science and public health made them both largely redundant within a few years. Nonetheless, the *Standard* expressed pride in the infectious diseases ward, which was certainly a great improvement on the shabby, prison-like structure it replaced:

> The new building which was designed and built by a local architect [W.J.T. Walter], builders [Fotheringham Bros] and other workmen, should prove a great acquisition to the city, for it will be able to give a splendid service to infectious cases.
>
> The new institution has been divided into two sections, for diphtheria and scarlet fever patients, while a portion of the old infectious hospital has been renovated for typhoid fever cases . . .
>
> A chain mesh wire fence erected in front of the entrance acts as a "keep out" sign, while a bell, which has been installed at the gate, will ring inside the Hospital.[10]

The new infectious diseases ward had forty-six beds, but only a handful were ever in use.

The opening of the nurses' home marked the beginning of two decades of virtually continuous building at the Warrnambool Base Hospital. The Hospital committee began this process with a skilful public relations campaign to point out the inadequacies of the existing buildings and the urgent need for their replacement. A typical article in the *Standard* was headed:

> HOSPITAL INADEQUATE FOR GROWING NEEDS
>
> Yesterday I made a tour of inspection of the Warrnambool Base Hospital—and witnessed a story of inadequacy, improvisation and congestion.
>
> Everywhere were examples of makeshift implemented by a vigorous board and loyal staff in efforts to cope with the rising tide of necessary expansion . . .
>
> Throughout the Hospital, in wards, storerooms, service and specialist sections, were numerous examples of efforts to "make-do" . . .
>
> At present 16 aged and infirm are in sections of the isolation hospital. In one female ward, which was intended to house 26 patients, there are now 35 patients, and in addition to this the outside verandah of the ward has had to be extended and walled to provide an annexe for extra beds.
>
> The men's ward, which was fitted to cater for 30 patients, carries 40 or over. Here again verandahs have been built into annexes to provide extra bed space . . .
>
> There is only one bath for the entire female ward. There is no shower at all . . .
>
> Most of the Hospital services, X-ray, pharmacy, pathology and outpatients are hopelessly inadequate to successfully provide services required of the Warrnambool Base Hospital . . .
>
> In the outpatients' section a waiting room with space for about a score of people had to cater for 34 to 40 people on ordinary days and anything up to 90 people on a clinic day.[11]

Similar articles appeared regularly throughout 1954, supported by deputations to Melbourne, reports to the Hospital and Charities Commission (HCC) and every other means of persuasion the Hospital board could think of. Finally, in November 1954, the HCC gave approval for the next stage of the Hospital's redevelopment programme, the construction of a services block to house x-ray, pathology, outpatients, pharmacy, physiotherapy and blood bank services.[12] The new building was only a single storey, but it was built so that a multi-storey building could be erected on top of it. The builder again was Mr E.S. Harris and construction was completed in June 1958. The pathology laboratory was equipped largely thanks to a donation by Dr Horace Holmes and completed in time for the arrival from England of Dr John Reid, the Hospital's first pathologist.

Aerial view of the Hospital, mid–1960s

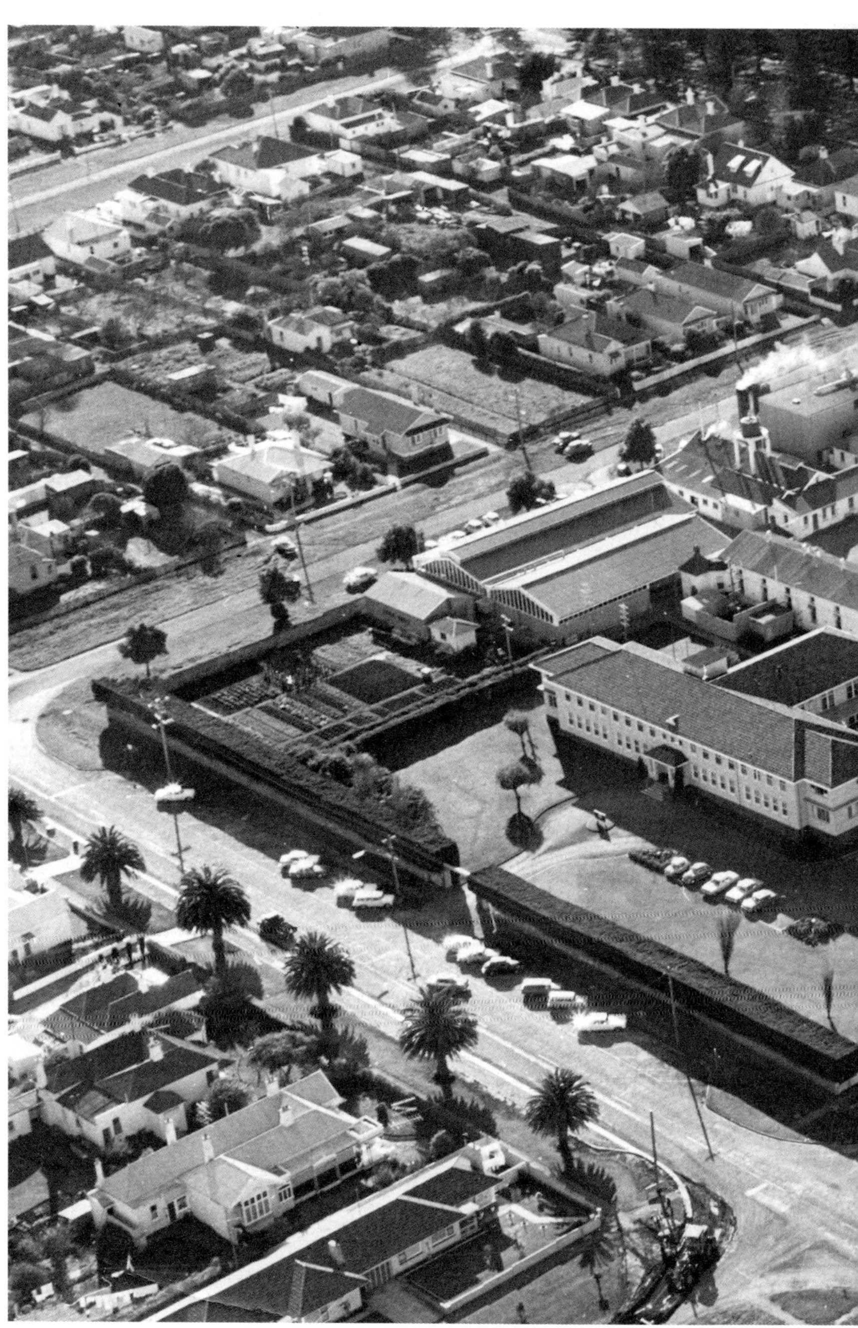

Immediately on the completion of the services block, Mr Harris's firm began construction of an amenities block, with a new laundry, staff amenities and mortuary.

Even before this was completed, the Hospital received approval to commence the centrepiece of the 1943 master plan, the multi-storey ward block which is still the core of the modern hospital. Again, E.S. Harris and

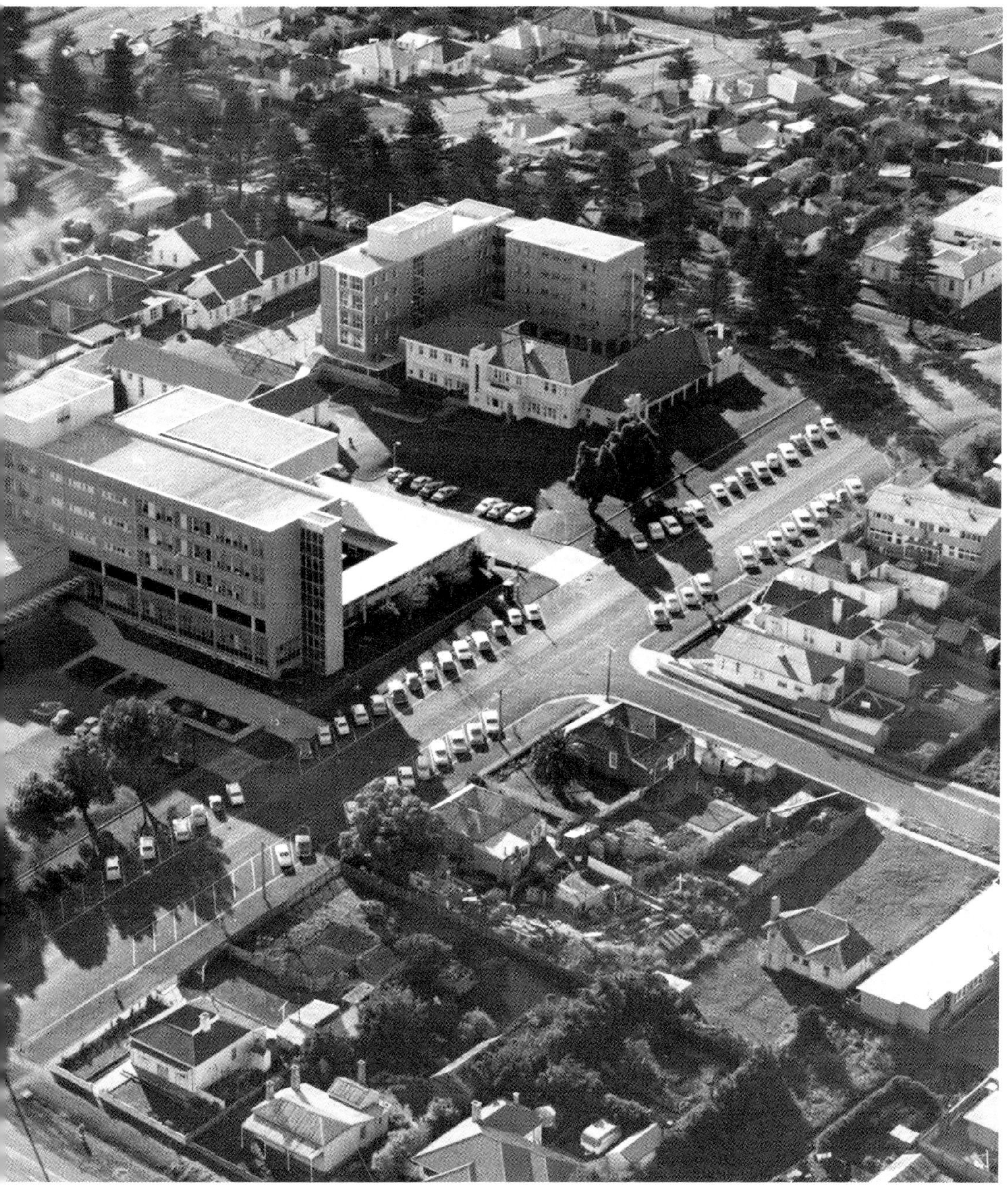

Co won the tender to build the new block—the tender being at that time the largest ever let in Warrnambool, at over £310,000.

The facilities provided in the new block included medical records, together with electrical and mechanical installations on the mezzanine floor, twenty-five surgical beds on the first floor, twenty-five medical beds on the second floor and twenty-three beds in the long-awaited new children's ward on the third floor. The original plans intended that the top floor of the new building should house a new operating suite, but, after thirty-nine plans had been presented by the architects and rejected by the medical staff, the Hospital committee decided that it might not be possible to build a suitable operating theatre in an elongated building.[13]

The new building was opened in November 1963 by Mr R.W. Mack, a man whose contribution to the rebuilding of the Warrnambool Base Hospital was probably greater than the official records indicate. Ronald Mack was a successful Warrnambool accountant, who was MLA for Warrnambool, 1950–1952, MLC for Western Province, 1955–1967 and Minister of Health, 1961–1965. Mr Mack said in his speech, "There is tremendous pressure on the Minister [meaning himself] and the Commission to find money to build in all parts of this state the type of construction that has been built here."[14] It was perhaps more than a

Outpatient medical service block, opened July 1958

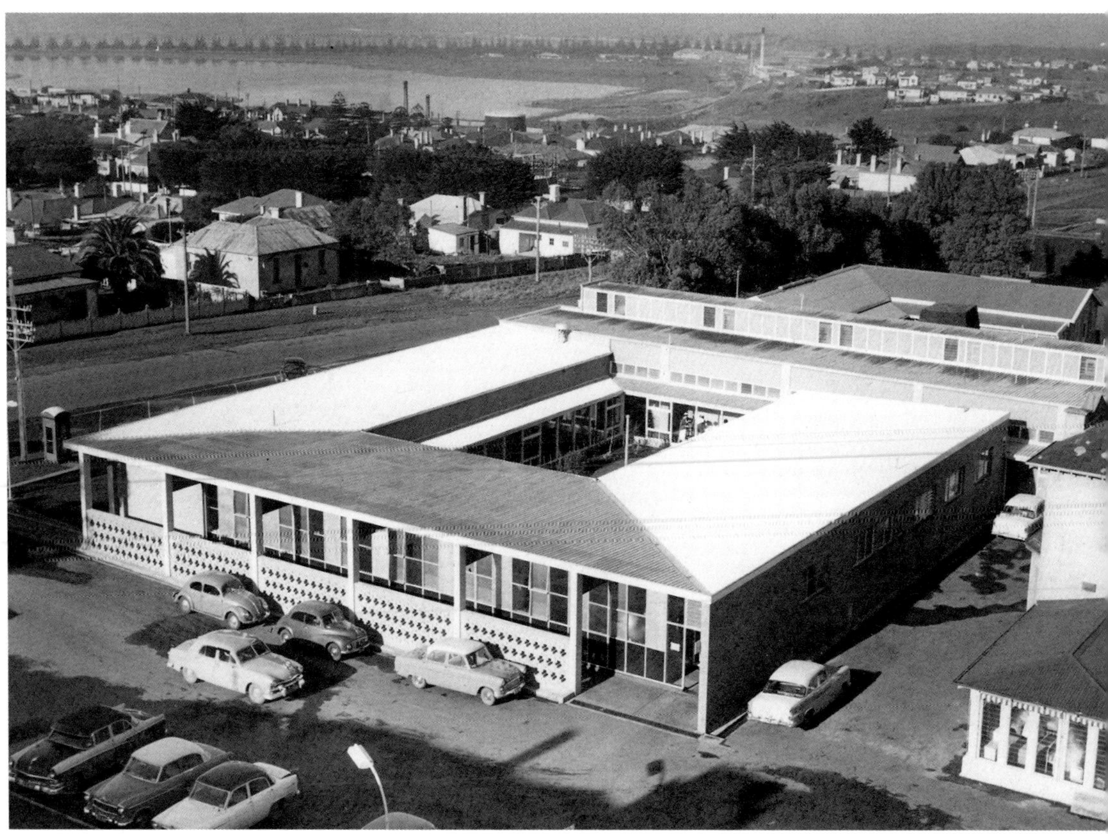

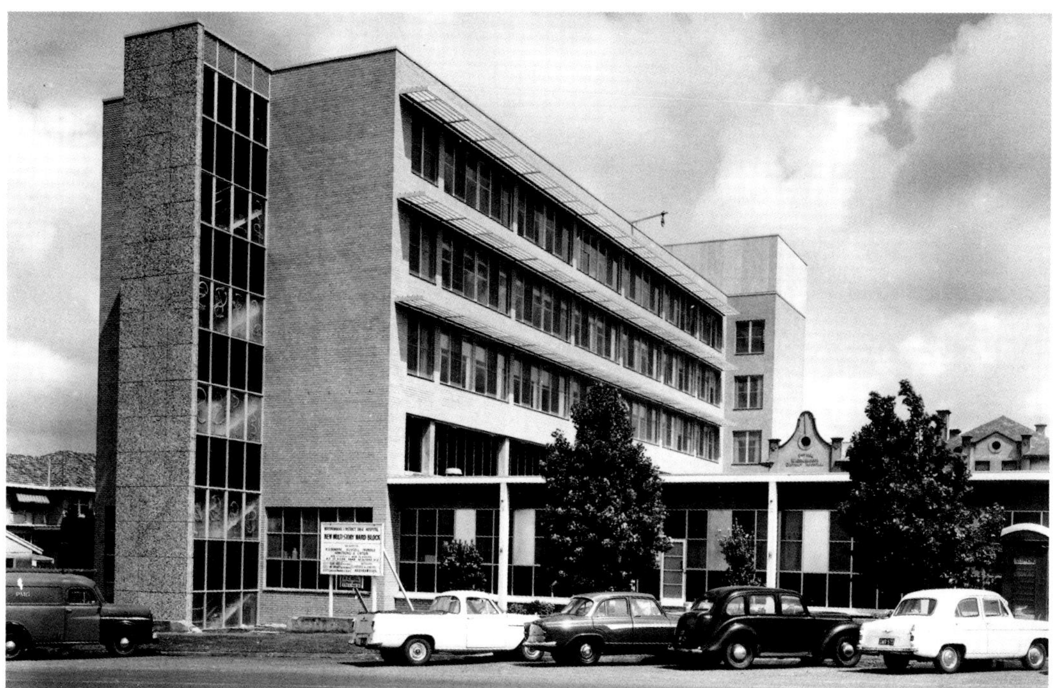

The multi-storey public ward block which was opened in November 1964. Note the older building at the entrance.

coincidence that the Hospital was highly successful in obtaining government grants for public works while a local man was Minister of Health. Mr Mack told the audience at the opening that the Warrnambool Hospital "would soon be second to none in Victoria", and he did his best to ensure that this happened.

From a historical point of view, it is regrettable that the construction of the new block meant that the original hospital building had to be demolished. This building, dating from 1861,[15] had been in continual use, but it could not be incorporated in the plans for the new building. It was a sign of the times that there was not a murmur of public protest at the destruction of this historic building—in later decades the Hospital would probably have been forced to preserve it.

Even before the opening of the main ward block, the Hospital began a large number of smaller projects. During 1964 and 1965 it was a hive of building activity—a report in the *Standard* in May 1965 noted that extensions to the surgical and medical wards had just been completed, the new theatre block was well under way, the first stage of a new boiler house was complete and the second stage had just begun, residences for the matron and assistant matron were approaching completion, as was a tutorial department for trainee nurses. Projects planned but not begun included a residence for senior sisters and new offices for administration and medical records.[16]

The new operating suite was built on the same level as the surgical wards and included two major and one minor theatres with rooms for anaesthetists, working areas for medical staff, and a three bed recovery ward. The time and effort spent in designing the theatre block resulted in a highly efficient unit. Unfortunately the boiler house was not so well designed as not enough room was left between the wall and the boilers to allow for easy replacement of boilers for servicing.[17] This may have contributed to the explosion of one of the boilers in July 1971. About sixty windows were broken by the explosion and one worker received minor injuries.[18]

In 1967 the Hospital completed a new casualty section, built in shell form at the same time as the operating theatres. The department contained a casualty operating theatre, casualty treatment cubicles, medical library, resident doctors' offices and a dental clinic. It was largely financed by a bequest to the Hospital by Miss Susan Kirkham, sister of Mr W. Kirkham, who had given many years of service to the Hospital as an honorary dentist.[19]

The opening of the casualty department marked the completion of the master plan of 1943, which saw the transformation of the Hospital from a small, outdated and inefficient assortment of buildings to a modern, integrated and functional base hospital. There followed a lull in construction activity for several years, and subsequent building has been to meet needs not envisaged by earlier planners. The first example of this was the intensive care unit which was opened in 1971.

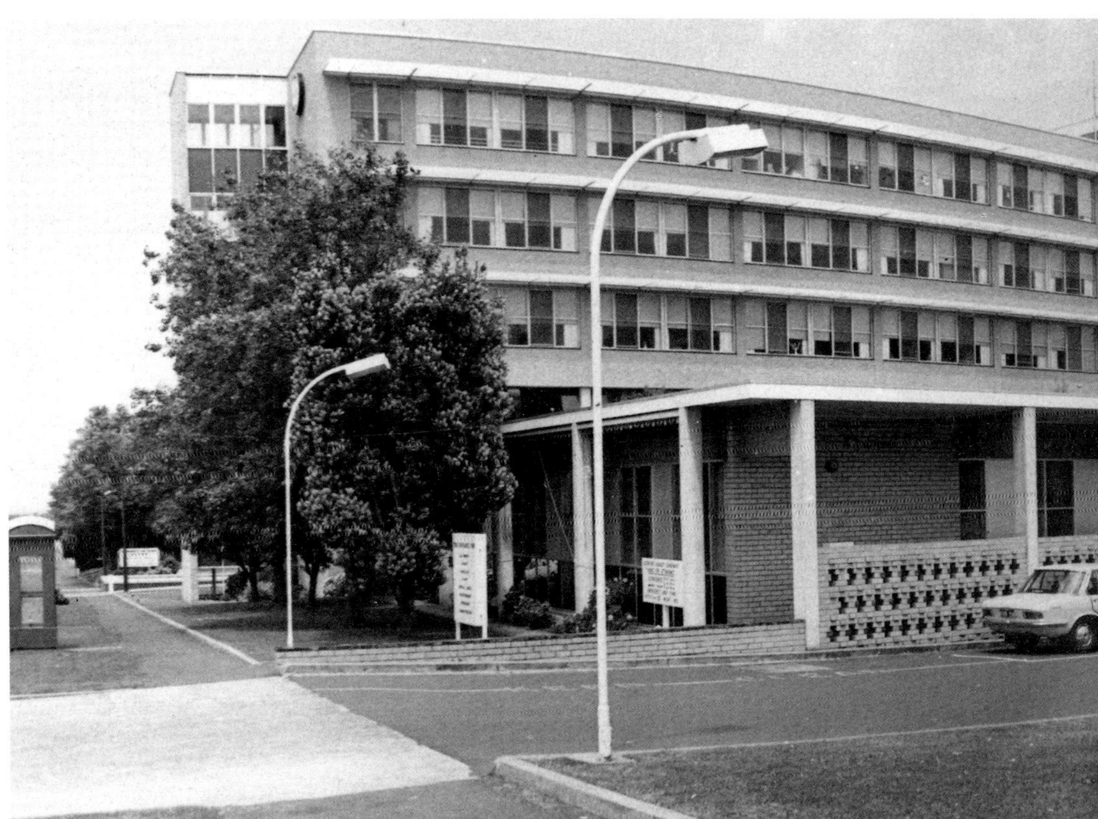

The evolution of intensive care has been the most important development in patient care since 1970. The concept of intensive care developed during the 1960s. Before this patients were sent back to the wards even after major operations, where they had to be "specialled" by the nurses. In 1965 a recovery room was built next to the operating theatres, but there was no allowance for intensive care. The key to the development of modern intensive care was the use of nasotracheal intubation to maintain the airway and ventilators to help very sick patients breathe. This was made possible by the availability of non-irritant plastic tubes that softened at body temperature.

The HCC approved the planning of an intensive care unit for the Hospital in July 1969, and Fotheringham Constructions won the contract to build the six bed ward at the west end of the main hospital block adjacent to the surgical ward. The ward was opened in August 1971 to care for patients suffering from acute coronary heart disease, acute respiratory failure and severe trauma.

The beginning of the 1970s also saw the Hospital take its first tentative steps into another major technological development, when it began to investigate the benefits of computerisation. The inpatient records were the first to be computerised, and the procedure appears delightfully

The multi-storey public ward block, with the outpatients and theatre block in the foreground.

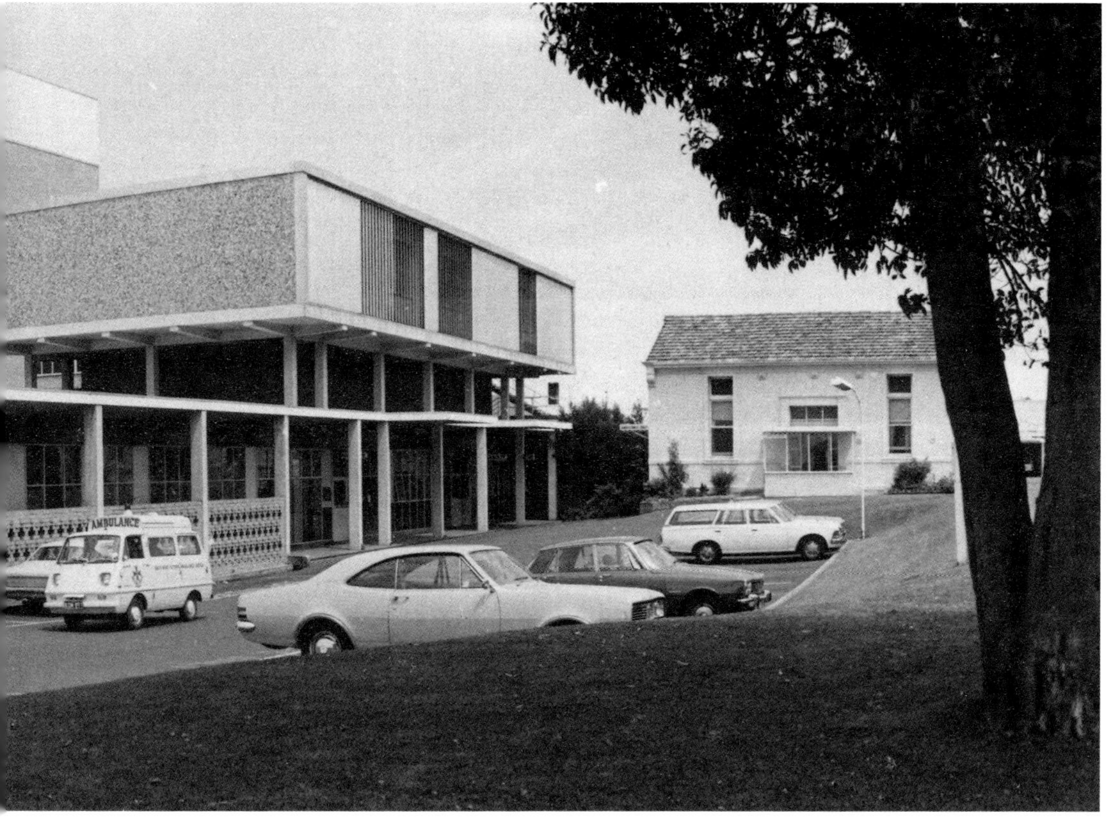

anachronistic: an office worker from the Hospital went to the Warrnambool Technical College once a week to prepare punch cards on the college punch card machine. The cards had to be checked carefully for accuracy as the college did not have a verifying machine. The records for each patient required three punched cards, which meant that about 1100 cards had to be prepared each month, ready to be sent by rail to Monash University's computer centre. In this way basic patient statistics were available within three days of the end of each month.[20]

The period 1945–1972 saw a transformation of the finances of the Hospital. In 1945 the Hospital's income was £19,918. Of this £4637 came from patients' fees, £4203 from local fundraising, £1766 from local municipalities as payments for the care of infectious diseases patients and the balance from the government grant. By 1972 income had risen to $1,294,953, with patients' fees coming to $650,000, the government grant being $550,000 and local fundraising making a relatively insignificant contribution of just $13,000. The size of the Hospital's operations had become so big that it was impossible to continue in the old charity hospital manner of relying heavily on local fundraising to support the Hospital's services. However, local support remained vital for the Hospital's massive building projects in this era.

The major building projects undertaken by the Hospital were financed primarily by government grants, but in most cases the Government required the Hospital to raise a certain proportion locally, normally about twenty per cent. For example, the multi-storey ward block was built in the mid-1960s at a cost of over £400,000, with the local contribution being £80,000. The Hospital was able to raise £30,000 from legacies, donations and past appeals (including the money raised by the original children's ward appeal of 1943) and the balance of £50,000 was raised by means of a public appeal.

The appeal commenced with a public meeting called by the Mayor, Cr P. O'Sullivan, in July 1962. Cr S. Price was elected chairman of the organising committee, Fletcher Jones was the patron of the appeal, and many leading Warrnambool business people became involved in various aspects of the campaign. Over the next few months the committee organised or sponsored an enormous variety of fundraising projects. George Swinton and Sons put on a fashion parade in the Town Hall at which Melbourne mannequins showed the latest metropolitan fashions, and Bruce Pritchard and Tony Benbow modelled a range of men's sports wear and suits.[21] The Caramut auxiliary raised £69 at a fete and baby show in the Caramut Hall—Gregory Surkitt was champion baby of the show and Elizabeth Hustler was judged the baby with the curliest hair.[22] Appealing to a different audience was the "international professional tag wrestling match" starring footballer Murray Weidemann, which was held in the old Y.M.C.A. stadium in Henna Street in November 1962, while the Apex Club organised a successful jazz concert in the Capitol Theatre in January 1963. A "Cherry Blossom" ball held in the Palais in October 1963 raised over £200 for the appeal. Lorraine Saunders

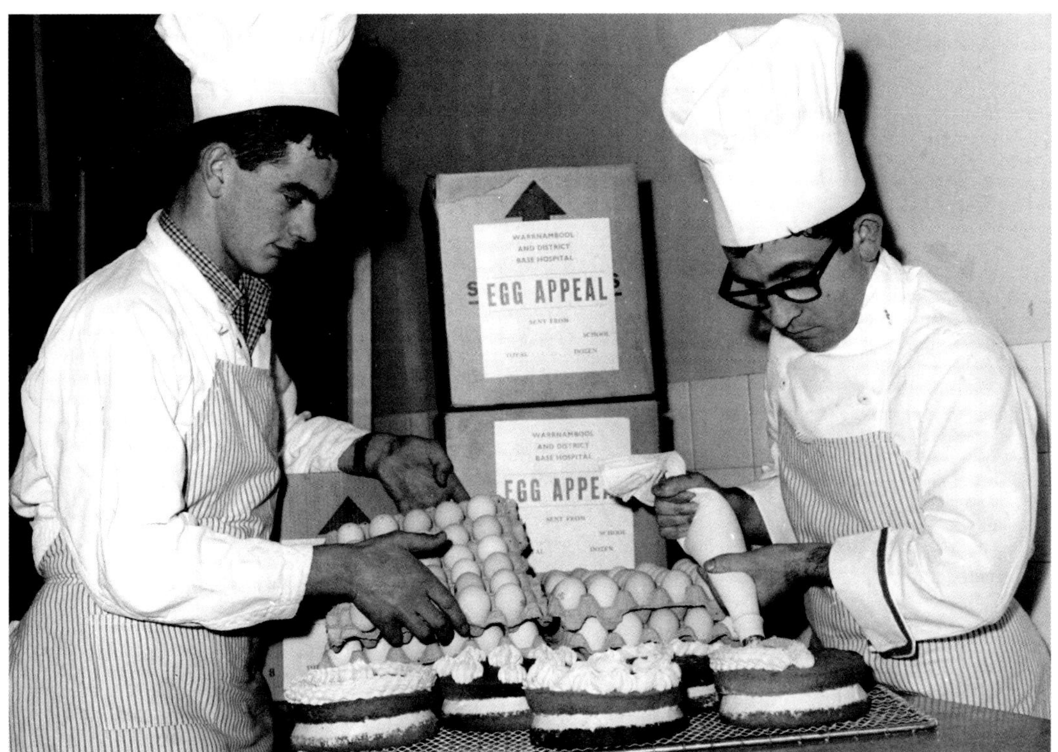

Egg appeal, September 1954

of Hawkesdale was chosen as "deb of the year", Nanette Shanahan of Warrnambool was "belle of the ball", and the compere was Malcolm Waldron (then an announcer with radio station 3YB).[23] These and similar events held through late 1962 and early 1963 eventually raised £51,637, with the largest single amount coming from the 3YB Hospital Sunday appeal.

While major appeals of this type were important for financing the major capital developments of the 1950s and 1960s, the local day-to-day support for the running of the Hospital came largely from the work of the auxiliaries. The post-war years saw a major expansion in the numbers, membership and role of the auxiliaries. Until the late 1940s the Red Cross auxiliary was the only auxiliary and its work was restricted largely to sewing and knitting for the Hospital. In 1946 the auxiliary had fourteen work groups, which attended the Hospital in rotation, mainly to sew and repair linen. The value of the auxiliary's work in that year was £40.

In the next few years the Hospital made a substantial effort to expand the auxiliaries. This was the period when soldier settlement was revitalising many country areas and the wool boom had given farmers unparalleled prosperity. Several new auxiliaries were formed in the surrounding country districts, including Caramut, Hawkesdale, Naringal, Nullawarre-Nirranda-Mepunga, Woolsthorpe, Grasmere-Cooramook, Purnim-Framlingham and Ballangeich. Hawkesdale was a typical example of the new auxiliaries. It was formed in March 1952 with Mr Lawson Glare as president, Mrs Colin Whitehead and Mrs Stan Baulch as vice-presidents, Mrs Richard Dawson as secretary and Mrs L. Sault as treasurer.[24] While the committee was largely representative of the old grazier families of the district, much of the support came from the many new soldier settler families.

The Nullawarre-Nirranda-Mepunga auxiliary was also founded in 1952, when Dr Buzzard spoke at the Nullawarre hall. Mrs Elsie Burleigh was the first president and Mrs Marie Lynes was secretary. The auxiliary raised money by catering at football matches and other functions, holding garden parties, and charging an annual subscription of two shillings and sixpence. In addition, the auxiliary committee divided the district up into seven areas and made house to house collections, a very effective fundraising measure.[25]

In the same period several new auxiliaries began in Warrnambool itself, including the Hospital staff, past trainees, and senior and junior auxiliaries. The role of the auxiliaries also changed, with the emphasis moving from providing goods and services to raising money. As a result, the auxiliaries spent more time organising fetes, raffles and other fundraising functions than sewing and knitting. A typical example of the new style of auxiliary activity was the garden party and fete held at Stan Baulch's property, "Rose Park", by the Hawkesdale Auxiliary in December 1952. The fete featured tennis, swimming, a baby show (winners Douglas McCosh, Arthur Leach

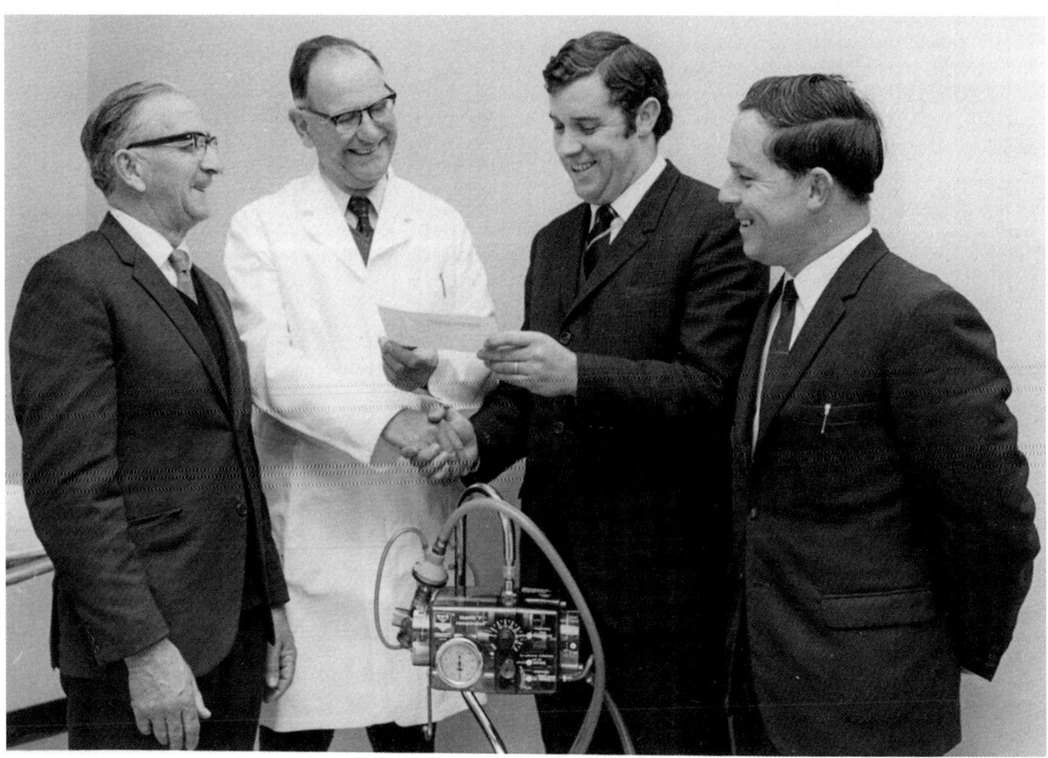

Mr D. Smith, Dr J. Reid, Mr N. Smith, Mr T. Mitchell, 1970, with a Bird 7 respirator presented by the Warrnambool branch of the Asthma Foundation of Victoria.

and Wendy Sharrock), a "Miss Teenager" competition (won by Jillian Adams), auction sales, lolly scrambles and peanut hunts. The fete raised £200, more than the entire value of the work of the auxiliaries just five years before.[26] For many years the Hawkesdale auxiliary held an annual book sale in Liebig Street.

Stewart Lindsay retired as hospital manager in July 1972. In his thirty years heading the Hospital administration he oversaw the complete rebuilding of the Hospital and a massive growth in the services provided by the Hospital. The average daily number of inpatients had doubled from ninety-one to 180, annual outpatient attendances had increased from 1000 to 53,000 and annual expenditure had risen from $30,500 to $2,500,000. The total staff of the Hospital had risen from 150 to 534. Stewart Lindsay had organised this growth with great skill and efficiency and he should be recognised for his primary role in providing Warrnambool and district with hospital facilities equal to any in rural Australia.

[1] Mirth Amelia Jamieson and Ros Lewis, "Helena Catherine Marfell", in Gordon Forth (ed.), *The Biographical Dictionary of the Western District of Victoria*, Melbourne, 1998, pp.94–95.
[2] *Standard*, 30 August 1945.
[3] *Standard*, 26 September 1952.
[4] Even inherently conservative bodies such as the Warrnambool City Council were infected with the passion for planning. See Sayers and Yule, *By These We Flourish*, p.254.
[5] *Standard*, 5 September 1944.
[6] *Standard*, 4 April 1944.
[7] The success of the appeal has led some later writers to assume that the new children's ward was actually built in the mid-1940s, but in fact a new ward was only completed as part of the multi-storey block opened in 1963.
[8] *Standard*, 30 October 1948, 28 November 1952.
[9] *Standard*, 7 and 10 October 1953.
[10] *Standard*, 12 July 1947
[11] *Standard*, 22 October 1954.
[12] *Standard*, 13 November 1954.
[13] Stewart Lindsay quoted in Ken Thompson, "History of Warrnambool and District Base Hospital", unpublished thesis in hospital archives, p.14; interview with Stewart Lindsay by Penny Forth, 27 August 1997.
[14] *Standard*, 18 November 1963.
[15] Some earlier hospital histories state that this building dated from 1853, but this is clearly incorrect as the first building on the present site was not constructed until 1861. See, for example, Thompson, "History of Warrnambool and District Base Hospital", p.15.
[16] *Standard*, 20 May 1965.
[17] W. Bedggood quoted in Thompson, "History of Warrnambool and District Base Hospital", p.15.
[18] *Standard*, 6 July 1971.
[19] *Standard*, 29 September 1967.
[20] *Standard*, 21 July 1970.
[21] *Standard*, 12 October 1962
[22] *Standard*, 15 October 1962.
[23] *Standard*, 3 November 1962.
[24] *Standard*, 8 March 1952.
[25] Notes by Mrs Marie Lynes, July 1997.
[26] *Standard*, 21 December 1952.

Chapter 14

NURSING, 1945–1972

The three decades after the Second World War saw both a radical transformation in the physical shape of the Warrnambool Base Hospital and a medical revolution which greatly reduced mortality and morbidity from many common diseases. While these great changes were going on in buildings and patient care, there was remarkable stability in the structure of both the nursing and medical staffs. The work, structure, training, and even appearance of the Hospital's nurses remained essentially the same in 1972 as in 1945.

The number of nurses rose steadily during this period, but nursing remained a rigidly hierarchical profession, with the various ranks distinguished by different uniforms, caps, veils and badges. The bulk of the nursing workforce was made up of trainees, who were almost entirely single women between the ages of eighteen and twenty-five. They lived in the nurses' home at the Hospital and had to observe strict rules on visiting, curfew times and many other aspects of their lives. Nurse training was almost entirely "on the job" and the work, in the early years of training especially, involved many menial duties. The senior ranks of nursing were filled with career sisters, who were almost all unmarried and lived their entire working lives in the confines of the Hospital. By the end of the period the pressures which led to the transformation of nursing in the 1980s were already building, but on the surface changes were minimal between 1945 and 1972.

One of the strongest features of nursing from the Second World War until 1969 was a constant shortage of both trainee and trained nurses. This was true of most hospitals, but it was a more serious problem for country hospitals than metropolitan ones. The Warrnambool Base Hospital had difficulty attracting enough trainees and equal difficulty retaining trained nurses. Frequently the shortage of nurses threatened the standard of patient care in the Hospital. There were many reports like this one from April 1948:

> The maximum service is being given to patients at the Warrnambool and District Base Hospital under extremely worrying circumstances, stated the manager-secretary, Mr. S.A. Lindsay, to the Board of Management last night. He was referring to staff shortages, a matter which board members discussed fully, without being able to reach a solution.

Matron D.A. Swinton in her monthly report drew attention to staff shortages, stating there had been numerous changes during the past month owing to illness . . .

The manager said there were about 60 members on the nursing staff, but owing to illness and the holiday roster there were not more than 50 nurses available at one time. The Hospital should ideally have 120 nurses in the seven major wards and the theatre

Mr Lindsay said that advertisements for nurses had brought poor results, and he had even advertised in papers of other states . . .

Mrs H.G. Marfell suggested that perhaps some assistance might be forthcoming if trained nurses who were married could be secured for part time, as was done during the shortages in the war years.[1]

The Hospital pursued many different policies to try to alleviate the shortage of nurses. In the late 1940s the Hospital had some success in recruiting trained nurses from England. The first three, Sisters Hilda Noble, Mary Westmoreland and Clare Brooks, arrived in May 1948, and several more groups came in the following years. Attempts to recruit nurses from European countries were less successful, as it was difficult for them to obtain registration and they found Warrnambool very isolated.[2]

From the late 1940s the Hospital also flirted with employing male nurses. In January 1947 the committee of management gave approval for the matron to accept male trainees, but added the rider that it believed that nursing was essentially a profession for women. There is no record of the Hospital actually enrolling any male trainees at this time, but soon after two male trained nurses from England were employed. These nurses, Mr T. Clifford and Mr J. Davies, came to Australia on free passages and arrived at the Hospital in early 1949. They commented to the *Standard* that "since arriving in Australia they had been treated more in the light of a novelty than anything else".[3] In March 1949 the committee of management noted that the English male nurses were happy in their work, but they found Warrnambool quiet after London and there was a fear that they would soon leave unless more interesting work was found for them.[4]

Several years later another English nurse, Mr C. Leonard, became sister-in-charge of the male ward. It is not clear how long he held this position, but Margaret Woodford, a trainee nurse of the period, recalls that Mr Leonard was among the first nurses at the Hospital to show an interest in rehabilitation. At that time there were two paraplegics in the ward, one of whom had been in bed for five years after a plane crash, and Mr Leonard encouraged the nurses in the ward to help them become mobile. He also started the rehabilitation of stroke patients by walking them with a nurse on either side.

By the mid-1950s the shortage of trained nurses was becoming less critical, but the Hospital still found it difficult to attract enough trainees. The main response to this was for senior nursing staff and administrators to visit local schools to talk with senior girls about the merits of nursing as a career and to encourage school groups to visit the Hospital to see nurses at work. Despite all the Hospital's efforts, the number of trainee applications did not match the level of vacancies until July 1969.

By far the greatest number of the Hospital's trainee nurses came from the district served by the Hospital. In contrast to the 1930s, few girls came from other districts to train at the Warrnambool Base Hospital. Although there are no statistics to confirm this, anecdotal evidence suggests that nursing was particularly popular with girls who grew up on farms in the district, as there would normally be no future for them on the farm and the bright lights of Warrnambool were a big attraction.

For many decades it had been generally accepted that hospitals provided accommodation, including full board, for their nurses. This had always been the case at the Warrnambool Hospital, but by the 1940s the number of nurses began to exceed the available accommodation. As a result, many nurses were forced to live in sub-standard rooms in the old isolation ward and other areas around the Hospital. Some local nurses were asked to return temporarily to their parents or had to live in flats in nearby streets. The committee of management believed that the most important step it could take toward attracting and keeping nurses was to provide sufficient comfortable accommodation, and this is why priority in the post-war building programme was given to the new nurses' home.[5]

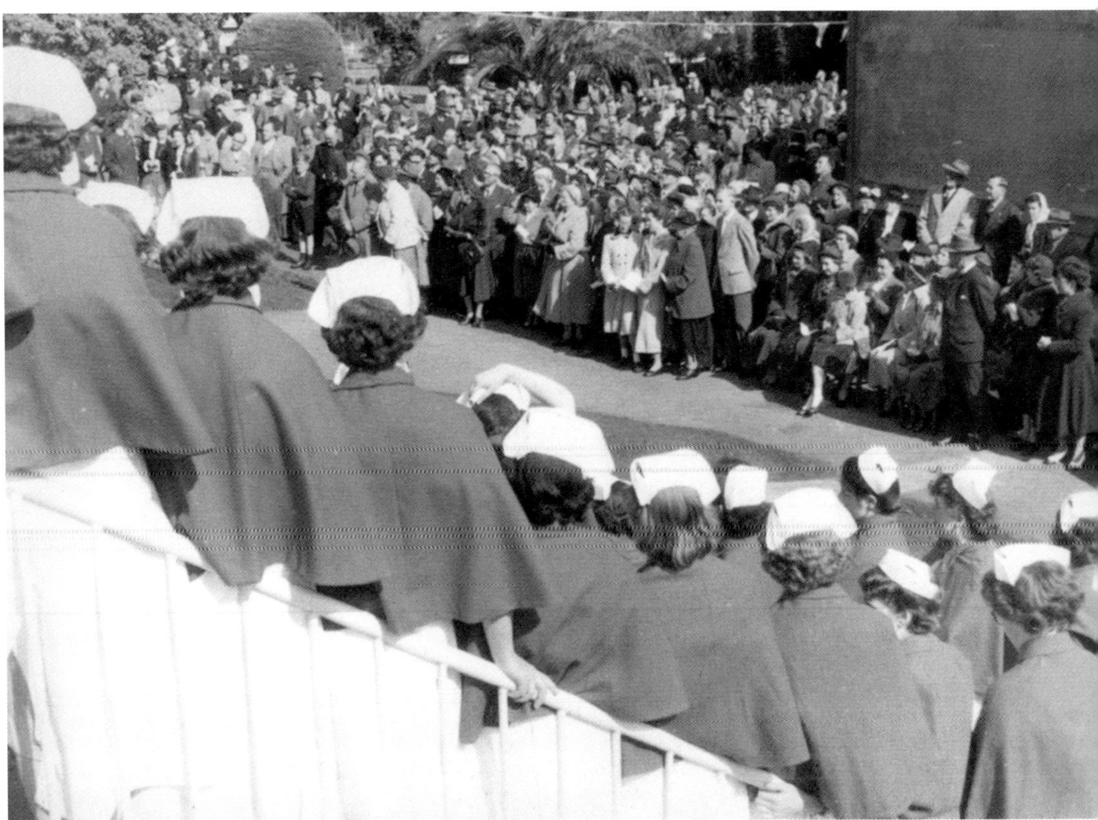

Opening of the new nurses home, 10 October 1953.

By the standards of the time, the nurses' home, completed in 1953, was modern and comfortable. As the *Standard* reported, "After their old over-crowded quarters, the neat individual bedrooms, ample toilet and laundry facilities and spaciousness of the new home are greatly appreciated",[6] and the nurses wrote to the committee to express their gratitude for their lovely new nurses' home.

Although nurses' homes appear anachronistic to modern eyes, the necessity for them was rarely questioned before the 1970s. It was thought that few parents would allow their daughters to become nurses if they had to find their own accommodation and were not sheltered from physical and moral dangers. A strict curfew, rules on visiting, and other restrictions were generally accepted as part of nursing life.

This is not to say that the rules were always strictly observed. Many nurses of the 1940s and 1950s delight in telling stories of their evasions of the rules. June Stewart trained in the mid-1940s under Matron Proctor-Brown and recalls that:

> We were never allowed out at night without written permission, but we had ways and means to beat the system . . . Filling our beds with clothing, putting on old wigs and clips on the pillow to make it look like we were in bed when we went out without a pass were some of these. It was usual to sign a book to get a pass, but if we wanted to be a little later we'd have someone to open the door for us and let us in at midnight or a bit later. Passes were rationed to two a week.

However, although the nurses strained the rules at times, they generally accepted the need for them and felt that the advantages of life in the nurses' home more than compensated for the restrictions. A group of nurses of the period recalled that, "For us, living in the nurses' home was like living in a family and we were very supportive of each other. And we still remain friends after all these years." The feeling of friendship and camaraderie was always very strong in the nurses' home and former nurses almost invariably recall their years there as being very happy.

The most important feature of nurse training in this period is that the Hospital was dependent on trainees for the greater part of its nursing workforce. Most nurses were trainees, with just a small number of qualified sisters to supervise them. Consequently nurse training was still almost entirely "on the job". In the early years of the period there was not even a preliminary training school and new trainees were immediately assigned to the wards where they learnt as they worked.

The new nurses were quickly given enormous responsibility. Margaret Woodford recalled that,

> After I had been training at the Hospital for nine months I was left in charge of the female ward. About thirty-five to forty patients were in it at the time and some of these patients were surgical. There was another girl with four months' experience, another nurse with three months' experience and myself in charge. Dr Buzzard came in to ask about whether a catheter

had been let off and I said I didn't know. He then asked, "How old are you?" and I said, "Eighteen."

The formal part of nurse training was the responsibility of the tutor sister. This position had been established in the late 1930s and was held through much of the 1940s by Sister Milne. June Stewart recalls Sister Milne as "a wonderful tutor sister" who worked extremely hard. The trainees had two or three lectures a week (in their time off), with the lectures being given in the board room by either the tutor sister or one of the honorary medical staff.

Over the period the formal part of nurse education gradually increased. The introduction of more complex equipment and the increasingly scientific nature of medicine required that nurses have a wider range of skills than had been necessary in earlier years. In 1948 June Stewart became tutor sister at the age of twenty-four and introduced a preliminary training school to give new trainees some knowledge and skills before they began work in the wards. Facilities for nurse training improved with the opening of the new nurses' home in 1953, which contained a lecture theatre and an office for the tutor sister. The time given to lectures and the resources devoted to nurse training gradually increased in the 1950s and 1960s, but nurses still had to attend lectures in their time off and the bulk of training was still "on the job".

The progress of the nurse training school received a setback in the 1960s following the appointment of George Coulson as sister tutor. Although he had had extensive experience in England and Australia, he seems to have approached his job with less dedication than his female predecessors. There were widespread rumours that he rarely gave lectures and spent much time working out of the Hospital. By 1967 the trainee's results in external exams were suffering and the board of management noted that the lecture programme was sub-standard and the whole plan of teaching needed to be completely reorganised.[7] Mr Coulson was eventually forced to resign and the position of sister tutor was replaced with the more managerial "principal nurse educator".

By the late 1940s nurses no longer had to work the extraordinarily long hours of earlier years. Nurses received a forty hour week in 1947 and, while many still began work early and finished late, most had two days off a week and were paid overtime. Although nursing pay was still very low, it has to be remembered that all nurses received accommodation and full board.

The nursing profession continually fought to reduce the amount of non-nursing duties—cleaning, cooking and the like—which nurses had to perform. This fight could never be completely won so long as nurse training was "on the job"—new trainees were not able to perform most nursing duties so they inevitably began with cleaning and washing, along with very basic patient care. The first confrontation between nurses and management over non-nursing duties in the post-war period came in May 1947, following the refurbishment of the isolation ward. The matron, Miss Langham, informed the committee that "the present system of nurses sweeping, mopping and polishing floors, washing and drying dishes, will have to cease as these are not a nurse's duty", and she had no nurses to spare for such duties. She suggested that a houseman should be employed to do these tasks.[8]

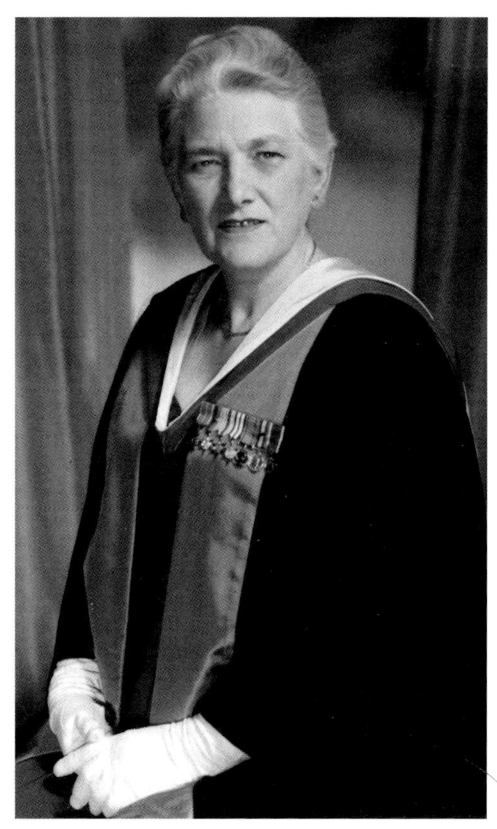

Doris Swinton, Matron 1948–64

Although the committee was not unsympathetic to the arguments of nurses, it took many years before the issue of non-nursing duties was fully resolved. Nurses who trained in the late 1940s and the 1950s all recall spending a lot of time with cleaning, washing, cooking and, when on night duty, even stoking the Hospital boilers. Until the new laundry was opened, nurses had to prewash the linen in the wards before sending it to the laundry "otherwise you'd have Bella [the laundress] in the doorway of the ward, fair bellowing."

It was on night duty that the nurses had to be at their most versatile. The most junior nurse on sponged, one of the night nurses had to wake up the next shift of nurses, and then at 7.00 a.m. they took in a cup of tea for the matron before they were able to go to bed.

The nurses of the late 1940s and 1950s have vivid recollections of their work in the isolation ward. The nurses were isolated as well, and the ward could either be frantically busy during an epidemic or very quiet. June Stewart remembers working in the ward in the mid-1940s during diphtheria, scarlet fever and whooping cough epidemics. She recalls that during a scarlet fever epidemic, the nurses in isolation were so busy that,

> We didn't have time to do all the children's hair properly so we seconded one of the older children to do everyone's hair—and then we had an epidemic of nits, because she had the nits! So all hell broke out as you could imagine. The poor pharmacist [Miss Lineker] was pouring stuff over to use every day—gallon flagons of it, and we'd put it through their hair and tie the hair in a triangle bandage overnight. She had a special solution made up that was very good—prior to that it was the old vinegar treatment.

Another recollection June Stewart has of the isolation ward is being on duty with Sister Miller, who was a devout Communist. While in the isolation ward the other nurses could not get away from Sister Miller and she used to give them pamphlets and harangue them about the evils of capitalism at all times of the day and night. They were tempted to spike her tea with a sedative, but in the end relief from political preaching only came with the end of their time in isolation.

The Warrnambool Base Hospital had five matrons in the period 1945–1972. These were Miss Proctor Brown, who retired in December 1945, Miss Jessie Langham, 1945–1947, Miss Doris Swinton, 1947–1964, Miss Barclay, 1964–1966 and Miss June Stewart, 1966–1982. Jessie Langham trained and worked at the Royal Melbourne Hospital and was with the Australian Inland Mission before joining the Australian Army Nursing Service in 1940. After service in London during the Blitz, the Middle East and New Guinea, she finished the War as assistant matron of the Heidelberg Repatriation Hospital.[9] She came to the Warrnambool Base Hospital with a tremendous reputation, but unfortunately her talents made her a target for other hospitals, and in August 1947 she was recruited by the Ballarat Base Hospital—the third consecutive matron at Ballarat to come from Warrnambool. Jessie Langham was described as "a nurse of the old school"; she had a "strong personality and an air of quiet, yet immense, authority".[10]

To succeed Miss Langham, the Hospital committee looked to another nurse with a distinguished war record, Doris Swinton. It is probable that the committee hoped that Miss Swinton's strong family ties to Warrnambool would help to prevent further poaching by Ballarat or other hospitals. Miss Swinton's wartime career has already been discussed in chapter eleven, and she returned to Warrnambool with a very high reputation. Although she was not an innovative or progressive matron, Miss Swinton had a talent for getting the best out of her staff and she gained the cooperation of nurses

Shaun O'Brien receives his Easter egg, donated by Fletcher Jones and staff from Sr Jean Knights (now Wallace) and nurse Janet Clague (now Houlihan), 1961.

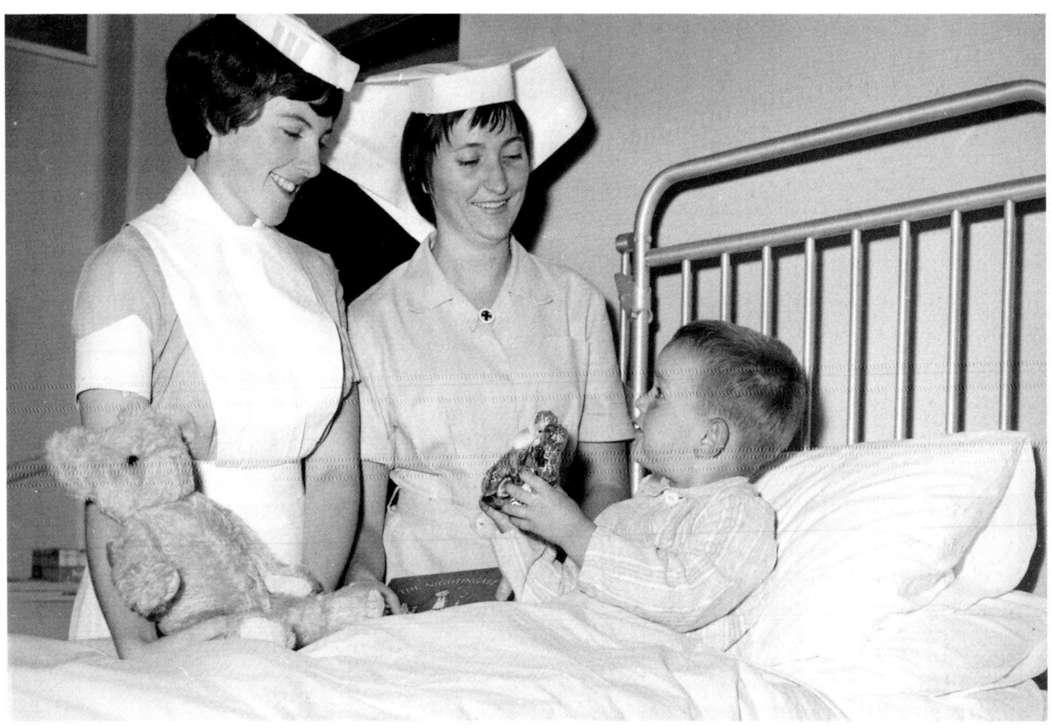

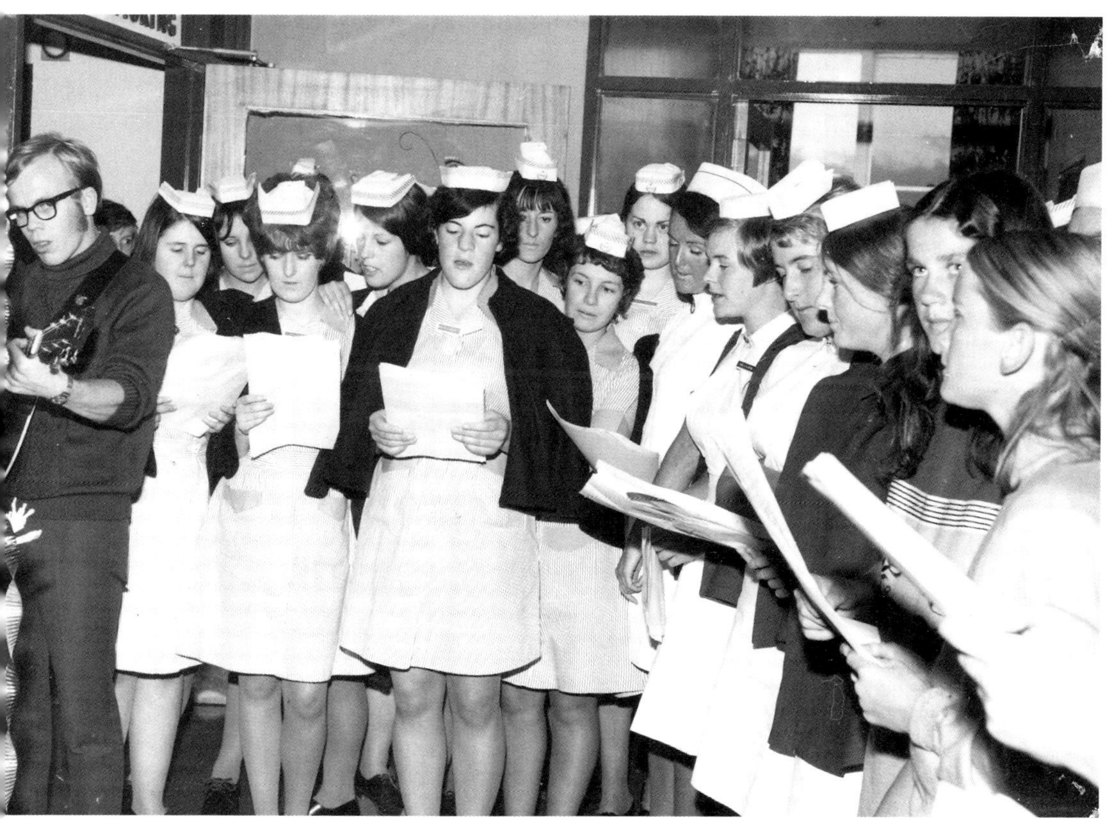

Nurses carolling outside the children's ward, 1969

and medical staff through her happy and outgoing personality. In 1963 Miss Swinton retired as matron, but she remained at the Hospital for several years as welfare officer.

Miss Swinton's successor was Miss D. Barclay, who came to the Hospital after seven years as deputy matron of the Mooroopna Base Hospital. Unfortunately her time as matron was not a happy one for the Hospital. The problems which had been developing with nurse education were rapidly reaching crisis point and Miss Barclay and the committee were unable to agree on the appropriate action for this and other problems. In February 1966 the committee of management asked Miss Barclay to resign, with one month's pay in lieu of notice, because the matron and the management were "not in complete agreement on certain administrative matters."[11]

To attempt to remedy the nursing situation at the Hospital, the committee turned to one of the Warrnambool Base Hospital's most distinguished former trainees, June Stewart. Miss Stewart had become sister tutor in 1949 at the age of twenty-four before becoming matron of the Portland Hospital in 1956. Her return to the Warrnambool Hospital marked the beginning of a new era in nursing at the Hospital and her term of office is more appropriately discussed as part of the next period of the Hospital's history.

By 1972 there had been little obvious change in in nursing since 1945. However, the increased complexity of modern medicine placed great demands on nurses and signs were appearing that radical changes would have to be made in the structure of nursing at the hospital. The 1970s were a decade of turmoil and change, characterised by staff shortages and a questioning of traditional ways. In the 1980s the issues of nurse education, pay and conditions, and the place of nursing in the health care system all came to a head and were only resolved after the trauma of the nurses' strike. By the end of the 1980s nursing had been dramatically transformed from the staid and stable profession of earlier years.

[1] *Standard*, 23 April 1948.

[2] Committee of Management Minutes, March 1961.

[3] *Standard*, 17 March 1949.

[4] Committee of Management Minutes, March 1949.

[5] For example, Matron Langham's report to the Committee of Management in June 1947, in which she "stressed the need for modern amenities in the new nursing home to attract nurses in the future".

[6] *Standard*, 12 November 1953.

[7] This paragraph is based interviews and Committee of Management Minutes, August 1967.

[8] Committee of Management Minutes, May 1947.

[9] *Standard*, 26 March 1946

[10] Anthea Hyslop, *Sovereign Remedies: A History of Ballarat Base Hospital, 1850s to 1980s*, Sydney, 1989, p.292.

[11] Committee of Management Minutes, 3 February 1966.

Chapter 15

DOCTORS, 1945–1972

There has never been a period in history in which there has been greater changes in medicine than the years following the Second World War. Long-established patterns of disease changed rapidly with many common diseases disappearing. A vast array of new treatments were introduced, and there was an enormous extension in the range of surgery and great progress in areas such as anaesthetics and radiology. Naturally this progress was reflected in the work of the Warrnambool Base Hospital. Diseases like diphtheria and scarlet fever, which had filled beds in the isolation ward for decades, became extremely rare, and the isolation ward fell into disuse and was eventually closed. The iron lungs for the treatment of polio and diphtheria patients with respiratory paralysis fell into disuse. The TB chalet opened soon after the war, but was no longer needed by the early 1960s.

Dr Irving Buzzard

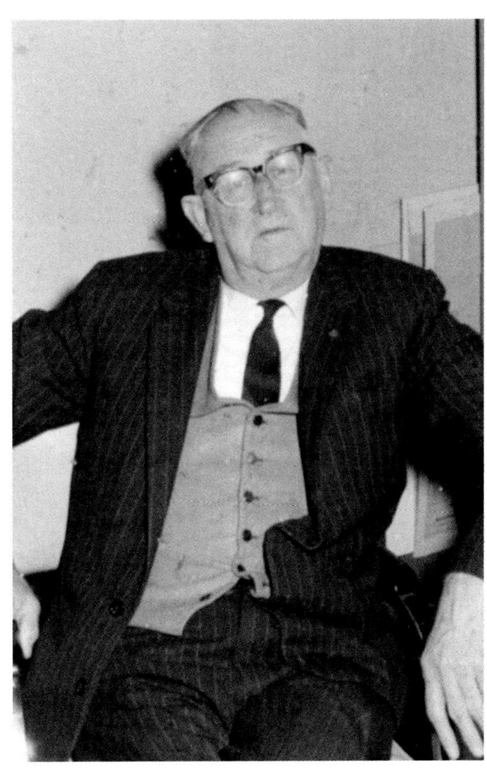

In many ways the work of the Hospital was transformed in this period, but strangely the structure of the medical staff, like that of the nursing staff, was almost completely unchanged. Until the very last years of the period, the medical staff was composed primarily of local general practitioners, whose work in the public wards of the Hospital was entirely on an honorary basis. The only doctors who were paid by the Hospital were the radiologist, from 1959 the pathologist, and the residents. Throughout the period the Hospital found it very difficult to attract residents and there were still only three in 1972.

Dr Les Hemingway came to Warrnambool in December 1958 when he purchased the practice of Dr William Ethridge in Liebig Street, on the site of the present art gallery. At that time there were about fifteen doctors in Warrnambool for a population of about

13,000. All the doctors were general practitioners except for Dr Park the radiologist and Henry Barbour the anaesthetist. There were three group practices—Doctors Brauer, Miller, Mouser and Longton in Koroit Street opposite Ambleside; Doctors Scott, Sobey and Beetham in the present Warrnambool Medical Clinic; and Doctors Buzzard, Gardiner and Awburn in the present Cambourne Clinic. Dr Hemingway recalls that,

> We all had appointments at the Hospital. I was appointed as a visiting surgeon on arrival. Dr Gardiner, the top surgeon, Dr Beetham, who was at that time doing a fellowship of surgery, was the second one and I was the third one . . .
>
> Back in 1958–59 we had Dr Miller, who was an M.D. but he could still take out our gall bladder or nail up a broken femur as well as anybody. Kel Gardiner was a master of surgery who could also deal with giddy old ladies and treat their heart failure. In other words all the specialists did general practice and all the general practitioners did a certain amount of what is now only done by specialists except that we all knew our limitations . . .
>
> Everybody did a bit of everything. We all used to fill in for one another. We delivered lots of babies . I delivered over 400 babies in my first four years. I removed thirty-four appendices in my first year . . .
>
> They were all honorary positions then. Everything you did in the Hospital was for gratis . . . Dr Buzzard was the obstetrician and Frank Mouser did obstetrics as well. Neither of them had a higher degree but both had a hell of a lot of experience. But everyone else did anaesthetics too. We used to do anaesthetics for each other. We used to have morning tea and chat about our cases—tap the brains of your colleagues and share notes . . . We all worked at the Hospital in the morning. We would either

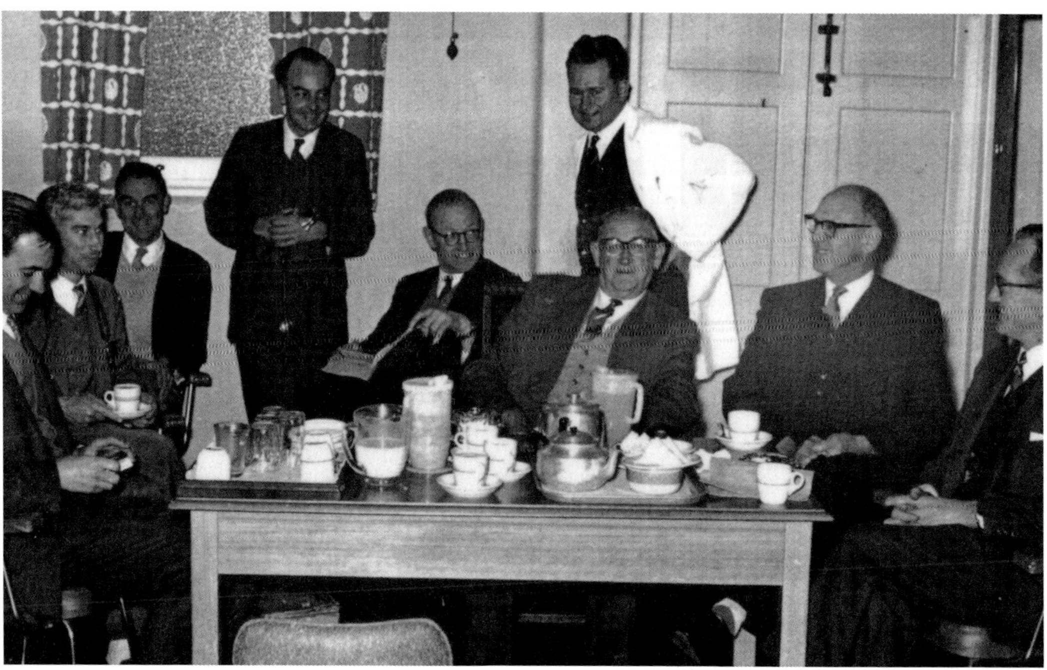

Honorary medical officers—having morning tea at the Hospital in 1961. Included in the group are (l–r): Dr L. Hemingway; Dr G.T. Awburn; Dr I.P.Q. Scott; Dr R.R. Sobey; Dr Irving Buzzard; Resident medical officer (unknown); Dr A.E. Brauer; Dr W.G. Miller.

> be giving anaesthetics for one another or for the dentists. Everybody was having teeth pulled in those days and everyone would have a few dental anaesthetics to give . . . Some did more anaesthetics than others. I didn't do a lot because I was a solo practitioner all those years. I had to choose between doing the surgery or the anaesthetics and I chose the surgery.

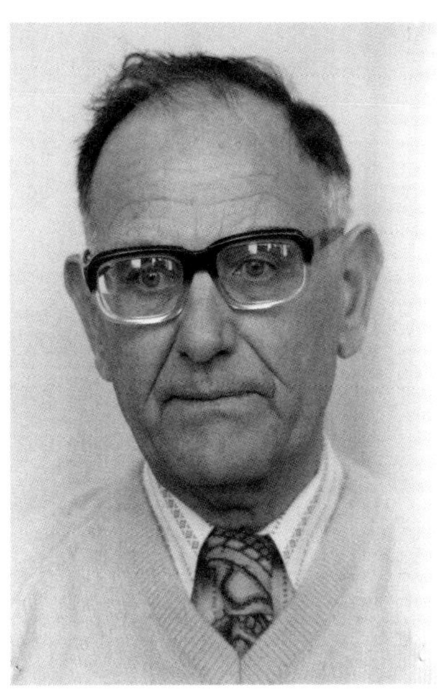

Dr John Reid, medical superintendent in 1966

Although all the members of the honorary medical staff were general practitioners, their appointments at the Hospital were as specialists and many of them did in fact have specialist qualifications. Thus, Kelvin Gardiner had a Master of Surgery degree and in 1962 received his FRACS, Dr Miller had an MD degree and Henry Barbour his senior anaesthetic qualification. The honorary staff in 1955 was made up as follows:

> Honorary consulting surgeons:
> Dr A.E. Brauer, Dr H.I. Holmes
> Honorary consulting obstetrician and gynaecologist:
> Dr I. Buzzard
> Honorary surgeons to inpatients: Dr C.B. Berryman, Dr J.K. Gardiner
> Honorary physicians to inpatients: Dr W.G. Miller, Dr W.R. Beetham, Dr R.R. Sobey
> Honorary anaesthetist and chest physician: Dr H.J. Barbour
> Honorary obstetrician and gynaecologist: Dr F.J. Mouser
> Honorary ophthalmologist: Dr W.R. Angus
> Honorary surgeon to outpatients: Dr W.N. Etheridge
> Honorary assistant anaesthetist: Dr K.W. Longton.

Dr Beetham, who was a physician in 1955, turned his attention to surgery and, on receiving his fellowship, became a surgeon on the Hospital staff; such moves were not uncommon.

At the start of this period, the only paid specialist on the staff of the Warrnambool Hospital was Dr Patrick, who had been appointed radiologist in 1938. Dr Patrick retired as radiologist in 1948 (while remaining on the staff as honorary anaesthetist until 1951) and was replaced by Dr Alex Park. The Hospital radiologists were not salaried staff but were paid according to the number of patients they treated, receiving more for private and intermediate patients than for public patients. The arrangements were eminently satisfactory for the radiologists—Dr Park earned £2300 in his first year in Warrnambool, an enormous income for the time.[1]

The Hospital committee established a second paid specialist position in the late 1950s with the appointment of Dr John Reid as pathologist. The search for a pathologist began in 1955, but it proved impossible to attract an Australian pathologist to Warrnambool, so from 1956 the committee began to explore the possibility of attracting a pathologist from overseas, offering first class fares to Australia and accommodation in Warrnambool as inducements. Finally in July 1958, with a fair bit of relief, the committee received an application from Dr John Reid of Edinburgh and appointed him to the position. He arrived in Warrnambool in April 1959 and over the next twenty years made an outstanding contribution to the development of the Hospital.

Dr John Reid graduated in medicine at Edinburgh University in 1933. He received postgraduate qualifications in public health and tropical medicine and spent thirteen years in West Africa before returning to Scotland as pathologist to the Peel Hospital south of Edinburgh. He recalled that when he arrived at Warrnambool,

> There were two technicians in the laboratory, Jeff O'Brien and Frank Clarence, who was due to retire. He [Clarence] had established the blood bank. The laboratory at that time was not well equipped and I was given £2000 to equip it. That didn't go far but I was able to get basic biochemistry, bacteriology, blood bank and histology equipment.
>
> At that time, the term "country hospital" was looked on as a dirty word, but Jeff O'Brien had good RMIT and Melbourne University contacts and we were recognised as a training centre for RMIT students doing a five year Diploma of Laboratory Technician. Towards the end of the five years the WIAE introduced a lower standard three year laboratory technician course which was good for us as we were able to get local people to come into the laboratory . . . after twenty years we had a staff of twenty . . .
>
> I was a salaried doctor without the right of private practice, but the Hospital and Charities Commission agreed to pay to the Hospital an amount of money into a private fund in lieu of the money I would have received had I been in private practice. This "special purposes fund" could be used for the development of the Hospital and the laboratory. We naturally upgraded the pathology department and with new equipment and technology we were able to do practically all the testing needed for acute cases.
>
> With all the money from the special purposes fund I was able to establish a central sterilisation department and installed one of these with high vacuum, high pressured steam sterilisers so that the sterilisation was done in minutes rather than hours . . . They were very new, very advanced and were a big advantage. I also installed Bird respirators in each of the wards and in the operating theatre for emergency resuscitation.

Stewart Lindsay believes that John Reid's achievement in building up the pathology department was "a near miracle".

Henry Barbour came to Warrnambool in the early 1950s as a young general practitioner with qualifications in anaesthetics. He had suffered from tuberculosis in his youth and this had led him to develop an interest in tuberculosis and other chest diseases. Dr Irving Buzzard appreciated the importance of keeping a doctor of Henry Barbour's ability in Warrnambool, and made him a generous loan to buy a house. Dr Barbour began a solo private practice in Kelp Street and was honorary anaesthetist and chest physician at the Hospital. In 1958 he spent a year at the Royal Children's Hospital to upgrade his anaesthetic qualifications, and for many years he was the only specialist anaesthetist between Geelong and the South

Australian border. As an adjunct to his role as honorary chest physician, Henry Barbour was appointed the government tuberculosis inspector for Warrnambool and District and, as tuberculosis became increasingly rare in the general community, this involved him in close contact with the Framlingham Aboriginal Community, where he established good relations with Banjo Clarke and other community leaders. As the only specialist anaesthetist in Warrnambool, Henry Barbour was permanently on call and his work load was unrelenting. He died suddenly in 1976 at the age of fifty-seven.

Dr Roy Angus was a member of the honorary medical staff for thirty-one years until his retirement in 1970. The Hospital's annual report for that year commented that:

> Although he practised general surgery, his main interest in latter years was Ophthalmology. He was a pioneer in the use of Intrascleral Cartilage Implant which resulted in cosmetically better artificial eyes (known as the "Angus operation"). The fact that a country practitioner can be a pioneer in specialist surgery is an inspiration to us all.

From the early 1950s the Warrnambool Hospital began to recognise the increasing specialisation of medicine by establishing regular clinics for visiting specialists from Melbourne. From 1950, Dame Jean Macnamara, Victoria's leading expert in the care and rehabilitation of children with polio and cerebral palsy, began regular quarterly visits to Warrnambool. During these visits she not only treated patients but also gave lectures to the nurses and community workers on the care of these children.[2] Dr Stoll began a regular clinic for cancer patients in October 1952, which he kept up for many years, and Dr Lesley Williams ran the tuberculosis clinic during the early 1950s until it was taken over by Henry Barbour.

In the 1960s, the Hospital began its policy of encouraging visiting specialists to establish private practices in Warrnambool. Although their hospital work was still on an honorary basis, the Hospital assisted them to establish practices, leased rooms to them on favourable terms and purchased equipment which was used for both their hospital work and their private practices. Thus in the early 1960s Dr Bishop set up an ophthalmology practice and Dr Rousseaux became the ear, nose and throat specialist. In December 1964 Dr Powrie became ophthalmologist, with the Hospital undertaking to provide reasonable equipment so that a service to the public could be established and maintained.[3]

The Hospital also encouraged doctors with specialist qualifications to join the established Warrnambool general practices. Two English doctors, Joe Brookes and James Rossiter came to Warrnambool in 1963 and 1964 respectively. Dr Brookes joined the Camborne Clinic practice as an obstetrician and gynaecologist, and Dr James Rossiter, came to Dr Brauer's practice in Koroit Street to be Warrnambool's first paediatrician. It is significant that even at this time both doctors joined general medical practices and, initially at least, worked as general practitioners as much as specialists. Dr Rossiter was appointed the Hospital's first honorary paediatrician in November 1964, with an agreement that all unattached public medical patients under the age of twelve should be admitted under his care.

Toward the end of the 1960s the committee and the honorary medical staff began to assess the future requirements for specialists. They agreed that priority should be given to obtaining a new ear, nose and throat specialist and that dermatology and urology were the most urgent new specialties to establish. At this stage it was still not seen as viable for Warrnambool to support full time specialists in these areas and the Hospital was looking only to obtain regular specialist visits. The first success of this policy came in 1969 when Dr D. Adin James began fortnightly visits for an ear, nose and throat clinic and was appointed honorary consultant otorhinolaryngologist to the Hospital.

The search for a new radiologist to replace Dr Park on his retirement was a good example of the increasingly active role of the Hospital in attracting specialist staff. The committee of management noted in October 1968 that Dr Park was due to retire in two years and agreed that a search should begin for a successor. The Hospital advertised in England and Australia and made direct approaches to possible candidates in South Africa and New Zealand, before securing the services of Dr Ted Rafferty.

An area in which the Warrnambool Base Hospital was somewhat slower to act than many other hospitals was in the appointment of a medical superintendent. In June 1946 the committee of management decided to call for applications for a medical superintendent as soon as it was able to obtain a suitable residence. At this stage the feeling was that the Hospital did not require a medical superintendent with a senior degree, but needed a "junior man with administrative ability".[4] By January 1947 the manager told the committee that the Hospital was not able to provide a suitable office or residential accommodation for a medical superintendent and that the best option in the short term was to continue to appoint a senior resident medical officer with extra salary to account for extra administrative duties.

After this there appear to have been no further attempts to appoint a medical superintendent for nearly twenty years. Eventually, in early 1965, Stewart Lindsay asked Dr John Reid, the pathologist, to become medical superintendent on a part time basis. The two men have slightly different versions of the conditions Dr Reid placed on acceptance. Stewart Lindsay recalls that Dr Reid said, "I'll handle it on one condition, . . . that I get no increase in salary".[9] Dr Reid's recollection is that he agreed "provided the doctors agreed to keep medical records properly".

As medical superintendent Dr Reid's greatest contribution was to convert the Hospital's primitive and inadequate system of record keeping into one of the most modern in the state. As part of this he initiated the Hospital's move into computerisation. He also greatly improved the control of drug administration and made many other important innovations to improve the running of the Hospital. All who worked at the Hospital during his term as medical superintendent admired his skill, energy and never-failing good humour.

One of the greatest problems the Warrnambool Hospital faced in the period 1945–1972 was a constant shortage of resident doctors. In the early part of the period this was due primarily to a nationwide shortage, but from the early 1960s it was increasingly due to the difficulty of persuading young doctors to work away from the capital cities. Until 1945 the Hospital had only had one resident doctor (when it could get one), but in December 1945 it was able to appoint two residents for the first time, as the end of the War meant that a large number of young doctors were discharged from the services and were seeking hospital experience. However, by 1947 the Hospital was finding it difficult to find even one resident and for the next twenty years there was an annual crisis when the time came to appoint new residents. For example, in 1957 the *Standard* reported that,

> Service at the Warrnambool Base Hospital was greatly handicapped by the lack of resident medical officers, the manager-secretary, Mr S.A. Lindsay, told a meeting of the Hospital board of management this week. Every avenue explored to date had failed to solve the problem, said Mr Lindsay.
>
> The number of medical graduates was inadequate for the demand and teaching hospitals . . . absorbed the Victorian graduates leaving insufficient for base hospitals.
>
> The board was told that no solution would be available for several years, since a decreasing number of graduates would be available each year.
>
> Honorary medical staff were doing all they could to give service, but they were all busy men and some inconvenience to the public could not be avoided, Mr Lindsay added.
>
> He was requested to attempt to secure at least one medical officer interstate or overseas, if none were available in Victoria.[5]

As the daily average number of inpatients in the Hospital during the 1950s was more than 150, it is hard to believe that the standard of patient care did not suffer from the shortage of resident doctors. For many hours of every day the Hospital had no doctor on the premises.

The accepted picture of a resident medical officer had always been an unmarried white male. Before the Second World War the Hospital had briefly employed a woman doctor and during the War there had been a married resident, but it was only in the 1950s and 1960s that the Hospital began to accept that it would have to broaden its ideas. Dr Alison Lukeis served as a resident for eighteen months in 1955–1956 and other women residents followed, although it was not until the 1980s that they became common.

In December 1957 Dr Buzzard, the president, told the committee that the only applicants for the position of resident were married and they had all accepted positions elsewhere, because the Warrnambool Hospital had no accommodation for married residents. He believed that the Hospital could not obtain a resident unless it could provide adequate living quarters for married couples. Following this the Hospital built two flats for residents, which relieved the situation a little. One of these was designed for married couples and the first resident to occupy it declared that he and his wife were very happy with it.[6]

By the end of the 1960s the graduation of the first students of the Monash Medical School alleviated the shortage of young doctors, but a tendency for doctors to marry younger made it imperative for the Hospital to provide more accommodation for married residents. Thus in 1967 the Hospital successfully sought HCC support to provide more flats for doctors and their families.[7]

From the mid-1950s the Hospital began to look overseas for resident doctors. In September 1956 the committee authorised the manager to make enquiries in England and South Africa, with the result that Dr Ray Laurence came to the Hospital as a resident in 1958 on a three year contract. This was a highly successful appointment, with Dr Laurence staying in the district as a popular general practitioner in Koroit. Following the conclusion of Dr Laurence's contract, the Hospital again enquired overseas for residents. Although it was unsuccessful in England, it did obtain the first of many Asian doctors to work at the Hospital. Drs Lim and Woo began work in December 1964, although it is not clear whether they had trained in Australia or overseas.

A further aspect of the Hospital's chronic shortage of resident staff in the 1950s and 1960s was that the Hospital looked closely at the training given to residents with a view to making it more attractive. For example, from 1963 each resident was attached to one of the group practices in town to give both guidance and experience. In late 1966 the committee agreed that the Hospital needed to boost the casualty and outpatients departments, as these were areas in which residents obtained vital experience, and the following year the Hospital began formal postgraduate training sessions.

While it is possible to chart the changes in the structure of the honorary medical staff, the slow rise of specialisation and the chronic shortage of resident doctors, it is more difficult to give a picture of the work of the doctors in the Hospital. In earlier days one of the most illuminating sources came from the reports of the occasional scientific meetings of the Victorian branch of the British Medical Association held at the Hospital. The leading doctors at the Hospital presented their most interesting cases at these meetings, and their case reports were printed in the *Medical Journal of Australia*. This meeting was attended by Dr Robert Southby, the president of the association, Mr Reg Hooper, Melbourne's leading neurosurgeon, Howard Boyd Graham, an eminent paediatrician, and many other leading lights. The cases presented by the Warrnambool doctors provide a fascinating picture of medicine in transition.[8]

The first case presented was by Dr Roy Angus, the Hospital's honorary ophthalmologist. His patient was a female, aged forty-seven years, who when first examined on November 9, 1949, had complained of frontal headaches with failing vision which was worse in the right eye. She was unable to walk properly at night, staggered in the daytime and suffered from shooting pains in the legs. She had suffered from "brain fever" at the age of six years. She had had six children, of whom two were living; the first was stillborn, the second died of diphtheria at the age of three months, the third died of pneumonia at the age of three months, the fourth and fifth were boys, who, according to the patient, were healthy (but both had since been found to react positively to the Wasserman test [implying that they were possibly syphilitic]), and the sixth child lived only a few hours . . . Her mother had died of exhaustion and her father, who was addicted to alcohol, had died suddenly. One brother was healthy, another brother had died before she was born, but the cause of death was unknown, and a sister had died of a tuberculous kidney.

Dr Angus then gave a full account of his examination of the patient, concluding that she suffered from optic atrophy of syphilitic origin, and instituted a treatment of malaria and penicillin. The patient was deliberately infected with malaria with blood taken from a patient in Mont Park hospital in Melbourne and allowed to develop nine major and three minor reactions before antimalarial treatment was commenced. At the same time she was given regular injections of penicillin. Dr Angus commented that this was the only treatment described in the literature to give the slightest ray of hope for the patient of avoiding blindness, as the pre-penicillin treatments for syphilis invariably hastened blindness from optic atrophy.

In discussion the visiting experts expressed approval for Dr Angus's treatment. They agreed that the case was one of congenital syphilis and that malarial therapy, accompanied by penicillin, was the appropriate treatment.

Another case which demonstrated the transitional phase which medicine was in at the time was presented by Dr Patrick, the Hospital's former radiologist, who was acting as honorary chest physician. The patient, a boy aged fifteen, worked as a farm hand:

> His illness had commenced with a "cold" six weeks prior to his admission to hospital in September 1949. He was treated symptomatically, but later became dyspnoeic and cyanotic, complaining of pain in the chest on breathing. His temperature was 102° F., and crepitations were audible at both lung bases. His condition settled down rapidly, but X-ray examination a few days later showed a condition very like miliary tuberculosis. On his admission to Warrnambool Hospital, examination revealed an emaciated, rather dopey boy. Except for a palpable spleen, no other abnormality was detected. Streptomycin was administered intramuscularly and intrathecally to a total of 51 grammes in ten weeks. Other treatment was symptomatic.

After sixteen days x-ray appearances were normal and the boy had gained twenty-one pounds. On discussion the Melbourne experts were somewhat sceptical of the diagnosis of tuberculosis, but the case is nonetheless interesting as it shows the extent to which doctors were aware of the presence of tuberculosis in the community and the use of streptomycin, at that time the latest antibiotic, in treatment.

Dr Kel Gardiner showed a woman on whom he had performed a lumbo-dorsal sympathectomy for hypertension, Dr Walter Miller a case of acromegaly, Dr Alex Park discussed the radiological signs of bronchiectasis and Dr Irving Buzzard presented a patient whose pregnancy was complicated by a benign vaginal tumour.

The introduction of penicillin, streptomycin and other antibiotics in the late 1940s and early 1950s was the decisive event in the development of modern medicine. This was followed by continual advances in all areas of medicine and surgery, with highlights being the introduction of polio immunisation, the evolution of intensive care, and the dramatic advances in the treatment of many forms of cancer. One development less publicised, but critical for progress in surgery, was the increased sophistication and safety of anaesthesia. In the 1950s Dr Henry Barbour was the only qualified anaesthetist in Warrnambool and most anaesthetics were given by general practitioners. Dr Les Hemingway has given a vivid picture of the anaesthetic techniques and equipment of the time:

> I thought the Hospital was good in those days even though we didn't have wonderful facilities. We had to make do. We had an anaesthetic machine we used for tonsils. . . It had a little electric motor in the corner driving a pump that blew ether which was highly inflammable down a patient's windpipe. Now that machine never ignited the ether, but theoretically it could have 100 times. Nowadays you wouldn't be allowed near that [but] . . . we did it safely. We just had to learn the limitations of our equipment.[9]

By 1972 the equipment available had improved greatly, but the Hospital still relied on one honorary anaesthetist plus the general practitioners to give anaesthetics.

For all the medical progress between 19745–1972, the structure of the honorary medical staff remained fundamentally unchanged. However, the years after1972 saw the long era of honorary service by the town's general practitioners come to an end.

[1] Committee of Management Minutes, August 1949, p.231.
[2] Committee of Management Minutes, July 1950, p.349.
[3] Committee of Management Minutes, December 1964, p.541.
[4] Committee of Management Minutes, June and August 1946, pp.380, 388.
[5] *Standard*, 27 April 1957.
[6] Committee of Management Minutes, June 1958.
[7] *Standard*, 1 December 1967.
[8] *Medical Journal of Australia*, 3 June 1950, pp.742–44, and 10 June 1950, pp.778–79.
[9] Interview with Dr Les Hemingway.

Chapter 16

THE RISE OF THE ALLIED HEALTH PROFESSIONS AND ANCILLARY SERVICES

Although the period 1945–1972 saw little change in the traditional structures of the nursing or medical staff of the Warrnambool Base Hospital, there was a rapid expansion in the allied health services provided by the Hospital. The existing allied health services grew rapidly and many new ones were established. Before the Second World War, the Hospital provided physiotherapy for victims of polio, but few other services beyond medical and nursing care. Most other allied health services such as social work, speech therapy, audiology and psychology were in their infancy, with only a handful of trained workers in the metropolitan teaching hospitals.

The story of the development of physiotherapy at the Hospital before the Second World War is unclear. In 1904 the Hospital engaged the services of a masseuse (as the earliest physiotherapists were called) on an honorary basis to treat the victims of the earliest polio epidemics. Subsequently physiotherapists were called on during each epidemic, especially the major epidemic of 1937–1938. The records are unclear as to the qualifications of the local physiotherapists, whether or not they were paid, or the facilities provided by the Hospital for physiotherapy treatment. But it appears that they were all women who worked at the Hospital on an honorary basis.

In February 1948 the committee of management noted that the visiting physiotherapist had been giving good service, and agreed that she should be paid on an hourly basis. The following year the Hospital responded to the rising demand for physiotherapy by appointing Mr John Grace as the first salaried physiotherapist. Mr Grace had experience at the Alfred and Children's Hospitals and was the first male physiotherapist in Warrnambool. He was appointed on a full time basis for six months while he built up a private practice, after which he was to work part time at the Hospital. There was a considerable delay before Mr Grace could take up his appointment, as the Hospital was unable to find suitable accommodation for him and his family.[1]

Mr Grace was the senior physiotherapist at the Hospital for many years, but as the demand for physiotherapy continued to grow, the Hospital found it difficult to obtain assistants for him. In the mid-1950s the Hospital employed a Miss Sveilis as a physiotherapist, but she was not registered in Victoria and, because of her overseas training, had no possibility of receiving registration. It is unclear whether the HCC approved of her employment, or how long she stayed at the Hospital.

During the 1960s the Hospital attempted to overcome the chronic shortage of physiotherapists and other allied health professionals by providing bursaries for local school leavers to study physiotherapy, occupational therapy, dietetics, and social work, on the condition that they work at the Hospital on completing their courses. This scheme met with some success, although in those days of full employment it was often difficult to attract suitable applicants for the bursaries. One of the holders of a hospital bursary was Paul Grace, the son of John Grace, who received a three year bursary to study physiotherapy with the obligation of two years' service at the Hospital on graduation.[2]

Speech therapy developed as a profession in the 1940s, but it was not until the early 1960s that the Hospital was in a position to consider employing a speech therapist. In October 1961 the committee learnt of the possibility of sharing a speech therapist with other hospitals in the region, but this scheme seems to have come to nothing. In February 1963 the Hospital granted a bursary to Sue Bartlett to study speech therapy, with a view to beginning services at the Hospital on her graduation. In February 1966 Miss Bartlett began work as the Hospital's first speech therapist.

However, the early years of speech therapy were far from easy. Sue Wasmer (nee Bartlett) moved to Melbourne in September 1968 and the Hospital found it difficult to obtain a successor. The *Standard* reported in that month that:

> Active operation of the speech therapy department at Warrnambool and District Base Hospital has been temporarily discontinued . . . a limited service is being maintained by a therapist from Geelong Hospital, who visits Warrnambool one day a fortnight . . . Mr Stewart Lindsay . . . said that the service had been in operation since January 1966 and there was a constant waiting list. He added that the 170 patients treated had come from Hamilton, Portland, Balmoral, Horsham, Terang and Cobden as well as locally.[3]

At that time two students were studying speech therapy with hospital bursaries, but it was not possible to obtain a Warrnambool-based therapist before they finished their courses in 1969 and 1970 respectively. Mr Lindsay said that "it was expected the district would provide more than enough patients to keep two therapists fully occupied". However, one of these trainees did not stay long, and Jan McKenzie was the sole speech therapist until joined by Liz Waters, another bursary recipient, in 1976.

Radiography was probably the most stable of the allied health professions in the period 1945–1972, but it still suffered intermittently from difficulty in attracting suitable staff. In February 1948 Mr J. Long came to Warrnambool as radiographer, but after fifteen months he took a year's leave of absence to travel overseas. On his return he remained for only a year, being replaced by Mr Larkin, who in turn stayed only a short time, being replaced by Miss Graham in January 1952.

By 1953 the level of work justified the appointment of an x-ray trainee. The Hospital committee specified that the job was most suitable for a woman, but a man would do if they could not find a woman. As it turned out, an eminently suitable woman did apply, with Judith Trees coming top in Australia in her final exams in 1955.[4]

Occupational therapy was one of the later allied health professions to develop in Warrnambool. In the years after the Second World War, volunteers from the Red Cross visited the Hospital for "diversional therapy". The matron, Miss Langham introduced diversional therapy in 1946. She explained to "Minette" of the *Standard*:

> The idea really originated as an interest for the patients—especially long term patients . . . I had seen the work the Red Cross workers did in military hospitals at Heidelberg and Moresby, where it was a great success in breaking the monotony for patients. Nearly all the metropolitan hospitals have Diversional Therapy workers now, and we are among the first large country hospitals to introduce them.[5]

In 1947 Thelma Dawson and Barbara Potter were the first diversional therapists at the Hospital. Miss Dawson had trained at the Heidelberg Hospital and Miss Potter undertook a Red Cross training course to become her assistant. Their work was entirely voluntary and consisted primarily of working with the patients making handcrafts such as scarves, slippers, toys, tea cosies and woven articles. This form of therapy was very useful in an era when many patients in the Hospital had long term chronic conditions.

Diversional therapy organised by the Red Cross continued for many years. The last mention of it in the committee of management minutes was in February 1964 when it was noted that Miss Macdonald had resigned as a volunteer therapist. It is not clear whether she was replaced.

By the 1960s, changing conditions made diversional therapy in the old style redundant. There were fewer patients with long term chronic conditions and there was an increasing number of patients with short term acute conditions. Basket weaving might be useful therapy for a teenager in hospital for months with osteomyelitis, but it has less relevance to a cardiac patient in the intensive care unit. The new profession of occupational therapy developed from the awareness that there was a real need for a more professional approach to the rehabilitation of patients recovering from strokes, trauma and other problems. The first occupational therapist at the Warrnambool Base Hospital was Jo Goodie in the early 1970s, but the story of the later development of this profession in Warrnambool, when the day hospital became an active rehabilitation centre, belongs to the next era of history.

While the Hospital worked hard to attract allied health professionals to Warrnambool, in many cases this was not practical in the 1950s and 1960s. In these cases the Hospital frequently began clinics and arranged for regular visits by practitioners from Melbourne or Geelong. For example, the first visit of an orthoptist to outpatients was in January 1963, when eight patients were treated.

The period 1945–1972 saw a rapid expansion in the ancillary services of the Hospital. The pathology department grew from a single technician performing a small number of basic tests to a major department with twenty specialised workers able to carry out many highly complex procedures. Similar growth took place in the pharmacy, while the Hospital established new departments of clinical photography in 1960 and medical records in 1965.

As the number of patients, number of departments, range of services and technological complexity of the Hospital grew in the decades after the Second World War, there was inevitably a parallel growth in the number and range of support staff required by the Hospital. From a basic staff of cleaners, laundresses, handymen, and kitchen staff, the Hospital came to need engineers, electricians, medical technicians and many other specialised staff.

Many of the great characters of the Hospital were long-serving members of the support staff. Rex Johnson worked at the Hospital for many years as an electrician and later assistant engineer. He recalls that,

> I fixed everything. Any ward would ring you up and you had to fix whatever the problem was. You just had to look at the machinery and nut out how to fix it . . . Only part of the work was electrical. I trained on the job and did courses on different things such as lifts. In city hospitals you can ring and get service mechanics out, but in the country you have to do it yourself — boilers, lifts, sterilisers and any equipment in the Hospital. I was taught to consider the Hospital as a ship with accommodation, a ship that takes people somewhere, and the Hospital engineer had to be the same as a ship's engineer and know a bit about everything . . . The lifts were probably the most common problem and people could be stuck in the lifts for ten minutes . . . We were on call every second week, all week . . . Most weeks we were called out each night, and sometimes had to stay up all night when the steam pipes burst in the boiler room . . .When I started there were only two engineers who could do call work, but later we employed plumbers, electricians and all could be on call.

Jessie Horwood was another much loved and long serving member of the staff. She described her hospital experiences:

> I was in hospital myself when I was about fifteen years old. I was in the old ward six—the female ward. I couldn't keep food down. In the morning I had to eat a very fine oatmeal, and then had to swallow an apparatus which drew samples up from my stomach every quarter of an hour till they had four samples. Things were different then and the food was very basic. For tea at night you'd just get bread and butter unless you had your own egg in your locker. We often got tripe for lunch.
>
> I started working at the Hospital about 1957 as a vegetable cook. My job was to peel and prepare the fresh vegetables . The vegetables were all fresh then and except for the potatoes, were all peeled by hand. I podded the peas, and peeled all the other vegetables too. We had a potato peeling machine for the potatoes. I stayed there for about four or five years, peeling vegetables and helping with other things and then I went into the dining room where I served the nursing staff their meals.

> We served the meals from a "hotbox" which was an electric trolley with space for four vegies and a meat, and for a cold sweet and a hot sweet. Meal times followed a strict ritual. The bell would ring and then everyone stood up for the matron and charge sister as they entered the dining room. The matron would then say grace and sit and then everyone sat down—nobody could sit down till the matron sat down. She would try and eat her meal as quickly as possible because she knew they couldn't relax until she was gone. When she got up to go, the junior near the door would jump up and open the door for her. I think they took it in turns to do this.
>
> I stayed in the dining room for about ten years. Then I was placed in charge of the domestic staff and had to see that the nurses' quarters and hospital wards were kept clean. I had to keep a watch out that the staff weren't hiding in the corner knitting. The doctors lived over the road in Ryot Street and it was my job to make sure that the flats were ready for the doctors. I would buy in some food, put out towels and soap as well as fresh flowers to make them feel welcome . . . We tried to make the flats as nice as possible to attract the doctors here.
>
> I remember one young boy who had cancer . He asked me for a special cereal—I think it was cornflakes. The Hospital kitchen had a different cereal. So I went across the road and bought him a pack of cornflakes. The next day I called in to see if he had enjoyed them, but his room was empty. When I asked the nurse where he had gone she said he had died. "And did he eat his cornflakes?" I asked. "Yes", she said, "He did indeed. And he really enjoyed them."
>
> There was also a little girl who had been kicked by a horse and wouldn't eat. So I said to her, "You tell Jessie what you would like to eat." And she said, "Boiled custard and hundreds and thousands." So I went home and made some boiled custard and bought some hundreds and thousands and gave them to her the next day. And after that she never looked back. Her father used to say to me, "Jessie, you saved her life!"

One of the areas of the Hospital which saw the greatest change between 1945 and 1972 was the laundry. Modern equipment and automation transformed the primitive laundry of the 1940s into a hygienic and efficient service. People who knew the Hospital in the 1940s invariably recall Bella Jenkins, the head laundress, as one of its great characters:

> Bella Jenkins was in charge of the laundry and she had a few helpers. They just had washing troughs and an old mangle, and they used to fold all the sheets by hand. If you went in there, depending on what sort of day it was, you could be well received otherwise you could be out very smartly. And they walked around, drenched in perspiration, and there was water everywhere. It was dreadful, really. Perspiration, the floor was wet and their faces were wet. Bella worked like any man in bib and brace overalls, bare feet mostly, and two of them would stand and fold the sheets like you did at home with your mother . . . They used to hang up the linen inside the laundry from lines hanging from the ceiling.

Although the laundry, like the rest of the Hospital, was transformed in the years 1945–1972, the true strength of a hospital comes from the quality of its staff. In this period the Warrnambool Base Hospital greatly expanded the skill base of its staff, enabling it to give more effective and more comprehensive patient care. Equally important was the dedication and humanity of its staff and the stories of Bella Jenkins, Jessie Horwood and Rex Johnson typify the strength of these qualities.

[1] *Standard,* 17 February 1950; Committee of Management Minutes, March 1950, p.307.
[2] Committee of Management Minutes, February 1969, p.379.
[3] *Standard,* 27 September 1968.
[4] Committee of Management Minutes, January 1956.
[5] *Standard,* 16 July 1947.

Chapter 17

WARRNAMBOOL BASE HOSPITAL, 1972–1998: AN OVERVIEW

The period from 1972 to July 1999, when Warrnambool Base Hospital officially merged with Corangamite Regional Health Service to form South West Healthcare, was a time of great change. As well as meeting a growing demand for a broader range of quality health care services during the 1990s, the Hospital board and senior management were required to respond to significant changes in the Victorian State Government's policies regarding the operation and funding of public hospitals. In addition, due to closures or the changed role of public hospitals in south-west Victoria's smaller population centres and increased growth in demand for specialist acute health care services, Warrnambool Base Hospital gradually assumed a role as the key health care provider for the wider region. During this period of considerable change and uncertainty, Warrnambool Base developed a reputation as one of Victoria's more progressive, efficiently administered and innovative public hospitals. External reviews of the Hospital, together with statements made by former patients, past and current administrative and medical staff and local medical practitioners, provide a consistent view of the Hospital as a well-managed institution. As a result the Base was able to respond effectively to major changes in patient demand and reduced government funding for public hospitals.

Two critical factors underlying Warrnambool's reputation as a quality regional base hospital were the general quality of leadership provided by the Hospital board and senior management medical staff and Warrnambool's general attractiveness as a regional coastal city. Effective, innovative leadership, particularly in the areas of financial management and industrial relations, together with Warrnambool's growth as a key regional provider of health and educational services, enabled the Hospital to attract and retain highly qualified medical staff, including specialist doctors in key fields. While community support, financial and otherwise, has remained important, it was not as critical as in the past. Flexible, innovative leadership was required to enable the Hospital to meet the challenges faced by all of Victoria's regional public hospitals during the 1990s. These involved responding to increased patient demand for acute care and outreach services, while at the same time facing major changes in the Victorian State Government's funding policies for public hospitals.

Effective leadership was required to enable the Hospital to react positively to such complex and potentially divisive issues as the introduction of casemix funding, reductions in government funding for public hospitals and the pressure to privatise or rationalise services.

Effective leadership by management in areas such as general staff reductions, contract negotiations with doctors and the privatisation of key departments meant that major changes were implemented with minimal disruption to the Hospital's operation. Faced with reduced government funding, the Hospital management was able to address these and other issues, such as the closure of Brierly Mental Hospital and negotiating redundancy packages with general staff. It also developed a range of outreach community-based programmes. This was certainly not the case with all of Victoria's regional base hospitals. Nor were some of these policy changes introduced without a degree of public controversy. Though becoming more culturally diverse, Warrnambool remains a conservative community, highly protective of its own. Major changes, which resulted from former Victorian Coalition Government's health policies such as the closure of Brierly and the Hospital's proposed amalgamation with Lyndoch Home for the Aged, were not generally welcomed. Yet these changes appear to have had little impact on the community's positive view of the Base. The view of Peter O'Brien, the Hospital's current director of management services, is that "The Hospital has . . . got a history of being better run than other country hospitals". This view is widely shared not only by other senior administrative staff, but most medical practitioners associated with the Hospital.

Dr Kevin Longton

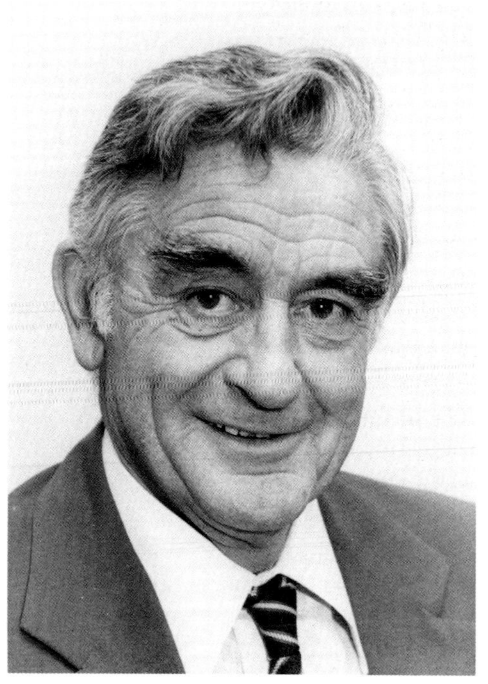

The role of the Hospital's board of management was to develop policy and be responsible for overseeing the operation of this large and administratively complex institution. While board members are not normally involved in the day to day running of the Hospital, there was at times a fine line between policy and management decisions. Prior to the 1980s the board appointed and reappointed its own members. However, in a change introduced by the Cain Labor Government in 1984, the Minister for Health now appoints members from nominations provided by the board. This change was meant to ensure that it would be more representative of the general community. In November 1984, following the expiry of their three year terms, Frank Lodge, senior vice-president, and Dr Kevin Longton sought reappointment to the board. However, while the then Minister for Health, Tom Roper reappointed Frank Lodge, Di Clanchy was chosen for

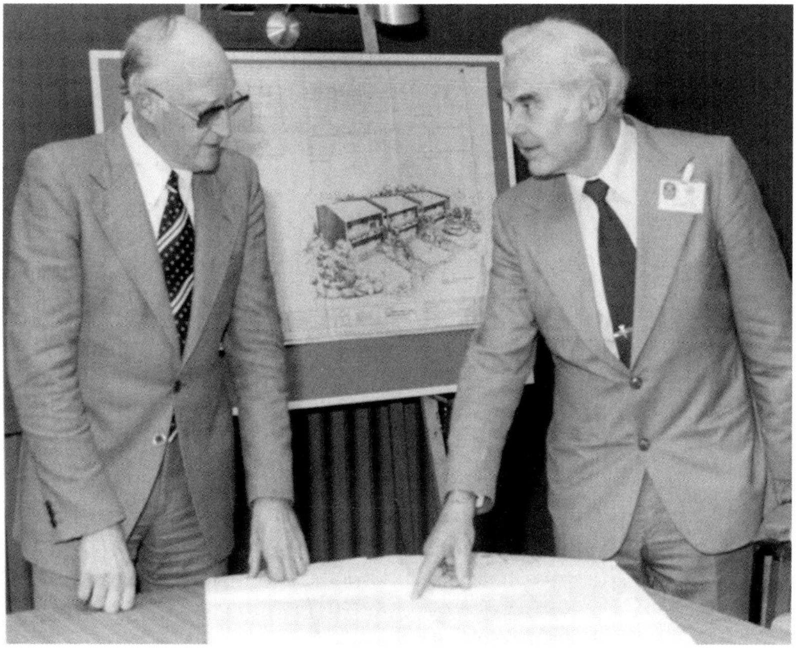

Mr Don Jenkins, board member; Mr Alan Matthews, manager, c.1980.

appointment over the highly respected local GP. The Minister justified his decision to appoint Ms Clanchy instead of Dr Longton, the immediate past president of the board, because her appointment increased female representation on the twelve member board to three[1]. To some extent this change has politicised the board. However, according to the current CEO, Andrew Rowe, this has not affected the board's working relationship with State Labor or Coalition Governments or the stability of the board's membership.

Current board members are aware of the need for ongoing education programmes to enable them to make well-informed decisions regarding the general operation and future direction of the Hospital. To be effective, board members need to do more than simply turn up and vote at monthly meetings. The board's responsibilities now include conducting the annual review of executive staff, and members need to keep abreast of complex policy areas such as privatisation of hospital services and casemix funding. According to the current president, Barbara Piesse, the Hospital board has been "able to embrace policies even though this has sometimes been very difficult". In short the board has been able to make necessary, but unpopular, policy changes such as the decision not to continue to admit non-acute aged patients, without public dissension on the part of board members. While potentially divisive decisions such as the proposed privatisation of the Hospital's pathology and radiology departments have been "hotly debated" by board members this has not resulted in the reporting of dissenting views in the local press.

Astute financial management is a key factor in explaining why the Base

Hospital was able to operate effectively during the 1990s, when the State Government reduced funding for public hospitals. This was principally due to the board's willingness to make hard economic decisions during the late 1980s and 1990s. During the 1990s with management committed to containing costs, the Hospital was able to develop new areas, particularly outreach services. According to the current CEO, in 1999 Warrnambool was "one of the few hospitals in the state...that has no debt". This is partly due to increased outsourcing and privatisation of services to reduce infrastructure and operating costs rather than to increases in the Hospital's annual income. As well as reduced State Government funding, the Hospital has no longer been able to draw on the Special Purpose fund. This former source of income generated though specialist doctors' treatment of private patients provided a significant source of funding for special equipment. This practice was discontinued when the Hospital privatised two key departments, a policy decision which the current CEO believes "more than adequately compensated for the loss of revenue".

Together with effective leadership and astute financial management, the good working relations between the Hospital's management and Warrnambool's medical fraternity has been important in explaining the institution's impressive performance between 1972 and 2000. The CEOs employed over this period—Alan Matthews, Peter McGregor and Andrew Rowe—appear to have enjoyed a good working relationship with the board, other senior managers and Hospital staff generally. Though individual medicos are critical of certain aspects of the Hospital's operation, when interviewed local doctors were generally supportive of the Hospital's senior management.

Due to the Hospital's sound financial situation and management's relations with staff, the impact of industrial disputes at the Base has been minimal. Even the Victorian nurses' disputes of the mid-1980s, which caused serious disruption to several of Victoria's public hospitals, had little real impact on the Hospital's day to day operation. For example, in March 1989, when nurses at the Hospital placed a ban on elective surgery, it only applied on the weekends when no elective surgery was scheduled[2]. The Hospital has benefited from having a harmonious, hence productive, work environment. According to Dan Dillon, the director of the Hospital's pharmacy since 1986, the "administration . . . have had great aspirations for the Hospital [and] been able to put them into effect". Interviews with local GPs and medical specialists closely associated with the Hospital generally support the CEO's view that "doctors have a really good relationship with the Hospital".

Yet it is also clear that something has been lost in terms of the attitude of employees towards the Hospital and the nature of the Hospital's relationship with the community. As with other publicly funded institutions, including universities, Victoria's public hospitals have had to become ever more efficient when faced with reduced funding from the State Government and requirements to rationalise services. As a consequence, as one former employee with a lengthy association with the Hospital pointed out, the Base may have become a "coldly efficient institution". Mr Richard Ziegler recalls a more relaxed time in the 1980s when Hospital staff put a great deal of time and effort into organising fundraising concerts and balls. Several of the doctors interviewed also referred to a time around a decade ago when the Hospital provided local medicos with opportunities for social and recreational activities.

During the 1990s reduced government funding and the privatisation of certain services resulted in a general reduction in the number of general staff. Yet while job losses which involved voluntary redundancies led to tensions, it is significant that the work of the Hospital was not disrupted by industrial action. According to Andrew Rowe, "there has been some friction" but probably less than elsewhere. Relatively harmonious working relationships between key groups responsible for operation of the Base helps to explain the Hospital's generally impressive performance since 1972. The view of one of the Hospital's current administrators is that previously the Hospital functioned as something of a sheltered workshop for many of the staff.

Prior to 1972, Warrnambool Base Hospital essentially served the people of the city of Warrnambool and its immediate region. The rest of south-west Victoria was provided for by a number of smaller public hospitals located in smaller population centres, including Hamilton, Portland, Macarthur, Lismore, Camperdown, Mortlake and Port Fairy. Although required to meet a common set of health care standards and government regulations, these hospitals did not function in a complementary way, providing a similar range of health services to the town and surrounding farming communities in which they were located. During the period 1972–2000 the role of the Base Hospital has gradually evolved from a general community hospital, which served Warrnambool and district, to that of the key provider of acute health care services for south-west Victoria.

As part of this process, in the mid-1980s the Hospital board made a critical policy decision to improve its range of specialist medical services. The board noted that, unlike other major regional hospitals in larger population centres such as Ballarat, Bendigo and Geelong, Warrnambool Base Hospital's medical staff did not include a wide range of medical specialists. In the 1986–87 Annual Report, the chairman commented on the "shortage of specialist practitioners in the area" and that "overcoming this recruitment hurdle will be the next obstacle to face".[3] As a matter of policy the board set out to recruit appropriately qualified specialists in the area of geriatrics, urology and paediatrics and to increase the number of obstetricians and anaesthetists. The success of the recruitment campaign meant that from the late 1980s, the Hospital has drawn an increasing proportion of its patients from outside its previous Warrnambool and district catchment area. As a result Warrnambool Base has increasingly been able to provide for patients requiring specialist medical treatment, who would formerly have needed to travel to Geelong, Ballarat or Melbourne. For the people of south-west Victoria there are clear advantages in accessing specialist medical services in Warrnambool. Less travel time is involved and waiting times for elective surgery in Warrnambool are considerably less than in most major Melbourne hospitals. Accessing specialist services in Warrnambool involves less disruption in the patient's family life and employment than if patients were required to travel to Geelong or Melbourne.

Because it had proven difficult to attract medical specialists from Melbourne, the board sought to recruit staff from overseas. As with other country hospitals, the Hospital's difficulty in recruiting specialists was partly due to the capacity of the Australian colleges of specialists to limit the supply of specialist medical practitioners. In any case even if sufficient numbers of qualified specialists were available, the problem remained of attracting them away from the major centres to work in regional hospitals. In 1986 the board authorised the Hospital's medical director, Dr Ian Carson, to visit the United Kingdom to interview candidates for positions at the Hospital. One of those recruited was a surgeon, Mr Brendan Mooney, who had trained in Dublin. Specialists were also recruited from within Australia. Two specialist pathologists were also recruited in 1988, Dr Mike Robson and Dr David Blaxland, and Dr Jim Barson joined the Hospital as a specialist anaesthetist from Melbourne's Austin Hospital. In 1988 Dr Mark Ivers was also appointed to the Hospital as a specialist psychiatrist. With seven new specialists in addition to specialists appointed in 1987, the 1988–89 Annual Report claimed that the Hospital "can now provide a true sub-regional referral service".[4]

While there was some opposition from Warrnambool's medical fraternity to the Hospital's policy of recruiting additional medical staff from overseas, most welcomed this initiative. One point of view is that the appointment of additional specialist staff had implications for the future income levels of existing medical specialists in Warrnambool. Although the board was keen to maintain a good working relationship with the local medical practitioners, it were strongly of the view that it was in the interests of the Hospital and patients to recruit additional specialist staff. The board's success in recruiting additional specialists was critical to Warrnambool Base Hospital's subsequent growth as the major regional provider of acute medical services. Having reached a threshold regarding the number of specialist medical staff employed in Warrnambool, it became easier for the Hospital to recruit additional medical staff who were initially reluctant to be the only medical specialist in their area in a regional centre. Had these specialists not been recruited, Warrnambool Base Hospital's capacity to provide a wide range of surgery and other services would have declined. In Australian hospitals surgery has increasingly become the preserve of specialist rather than general surgeons, requiring an increasing level of accredited expertise.

Warrnambool Base Hospital's role as a regional health provider was also due to a gradual reduction in the services provided by other hospitals in south-west Victoria. Hospitals in smaller population centres such as Port Fairy, Macarthur, Camperdown and Mortlake were generally unable to attract the specialist medical staff required to continue to function as autonomous hospitals. To a lesser extent this is also true of the hospitals located in the region's medium-sized population centres such as Hamilton and Portland. Serving populations of less than 10,000, Hamilton and Portland Hospitals cannot offer the same range of medical services as hospitals located in larger population centres such as Warrnambool, Shepparton and Bendigo. This change has been particularly significant for Hamilton Base Hospital, which was formerly recognised as the leading hospital in south-west Victoria.

The broadening of the range of services offered in Warrnambool together with reduced medical services available in other centres resulted in the growth of Warrnambool Base Hospital. Whereas formerly residents of the Warrnambool district requiring specialist medical attention often needed to travel to Melbourne, there are now some Melbourne residents, faced with a lengthy waiting time for elective surgery, who have their operations in Warrnambool. However it is not the board's policy to encourage this trend to the extent that it would result in a reduced level of service for local residents. The current catchment area of South West Healthcare varies according to the service being provided. In the case of psychiatric services, there is an estimated catchment population of 103,000, with service being provided in Warrnambool, Camperdown, Hamilton and Portland. In terms of the traditional hospital health services the catchment areas are much smaller. In the case of more specialised medical services the location for treatment now depends on the level of treatment required. For example, a general surgeon at the Hamilton Hospital may treat a Hamilton resident in need of an orthopaedic operation. However if the treatment is more complex it may be deemed appropriate to have the patient treated by an orthopaedic specialist located at Warrnambool, or possibly referred to a surgeon in Melbourne.

In the short term it seems unlikely that the board of South West Health Services will repeat its overseas recruitment campaign to attract additional or replacement specialist medical staff. This is partly due to a restructuring of hospital services in Melbourne during the 1990s, which resulted in the closure of several inner city hospitals and the opening of new hospitals in the outer suburbs. As a result the prospect of practising in a major regional centre such as Warrnambool became a more attractive option for Melbourne-based medical specialists. In addition recent developments in information technology have reduced the isolation of medical professionals practising outside the metropolitan area. Sophisticated information technology now allows medical practitioners located in Warrnambool to have direct access to the latest developments in their fields. A number of medical staff at the

Warrnambool Base Hospital have appointments to St Vincent's Hospital in Melbourne, which they visit on a weekly or fortnightly basis to keep abreast of recent developments in medical science.

Partly as a result of the growth in the number of and range of expertise of medical staff at the Warrnambool Base Hospital, the patient workload of the Hospital has more than doubled over the past twenty years. Although there has been an extensive building programme over this period, this has not resulted in a significant increase in the number of patient beds. This is because the average the length of stay of patients at the Hospital has halved since the early 1970s. Due to the increased cost of maintaining non-acute patients in hospital and the development of support services, an increasing proportion of the Hospital's patients are now cared for in their homes. The impressive growth in the range of services offered by the Hospital would not have been possible if the average length of stay of patients in hospital had not been significantly reduced. For example, in 1983–84 Warrnambool Base Hospital treated 5834 inpatients with an average length of stay of nine days. In 1998–99 the Hospital treated 13,000 patients with an average length of stay of three and a half days. This trend is continuing.

Another factor which has contributed to a reduced demand for Hospital beds is the change in the Hospital's aged care policy which occurred in the mid-1980s. Until this time many of Warrnambool's older residents, although still capable of living independent lives, albeit with assistance, sought admittance to nursing homes such as Lyndoch or to a bed at the Base. This was partly due to a general lack of support services to enable older people who were not chronically ill to remain in their homes. During the 1990s changes in the Victorian State Government Health Department policies and the Commonwealth aged care assessment requirements made it more difficult to gain admittance to a nursing home. In Warrnambool, as in other centres, the emphasis has been to provide an increased range of support services to enable non acute, aged patients to remain in their own homes as long as possible. The current situation is now quite different from that which existed up to the mid-1980s, when the Hospital provided beds to people who were elderly but not chronically sick. It was common for the Hospital to provide beds for up to fifteen patients who were waiting to be admitted to nursing homes.

Another major challenge facing the Hospital over the past twenty-eight years has been to provide high quality modern equipment to support the work of the Hospital, including new health services administered by the Base Hospital. One solution to meeting the high cost involved in replacing expensive medical equipment has been to privatise facets of the Hospital's operation. The two major diagnostic departments privatised at the Warrnambool Base Hospital were pathology and radiology. The Hospital Board's decision to put the Hospital's radiology services out to private tender was somewhat controversial. Radiology services had been provided by Western District Radiology Services who then established private rooms in opposition to the Hospital's own radiology service. As a consequence the revenue to the Hospital's radiology services declined and by the mid-1980s the Hospital had a sub-standard, somewhat rundown radiology department. The public announcement that the contract for the Hospital's radiology services had been awarded to outside tenderers Drs Rohan Wright and Paul Walker caused quite a ripple amongst Warrnambool's medical establishment. Drs Wright and Walker, who subsequently formed an arrangement with the Mayne Nickless Group, lease space within the Hospital, and are responsible for the employment of staff, the purchase and maintenance of equipment and the general operation of radiology services within the Hospital. This group has spent around three million dollars on new equipment. Western District Radiology Services subsequently located to St John of God, a Catholic hospital located in Warrnambool, and now provides an alternative to the Warrnambool Base Hospital's radiology service. According to Andrew Rowe, Warrnambool is fortunate to have two radiology services as competition ensures that patients receive superior, more cost efficient service.

Privatisation of certain services is but one of several policies that the former State Coalition Government required Victoria's public hospitals to adopt in the interest of increased efficiency. Prior to the 1990s public hospitals such as Warrnambool Base Hospital received State Government funding on a historic basis. This meant public hospitals received a similar allocation to that of the previous year with an allowance for salary increases and inflation but also possible reductions in funding.

In 1993 the Minister for Health, Marie Tehan, introduced the casemix funding formula which sought to address significant anomalies in the funding formula. Under the historical model two hospitals could receive approximately the same allocation from the State Government, though one might have double the workload of the other and a higher proportion of more complex, therefore more expensive, cases. Casemix funding provided for hospitals to be paid for set procedures under a code developed by the State Government, according to a set level of funding for services provided. The casemix formula also enabled the State Government to cap Warrnambool Hospital's workload. For example, if the Hospital performed more hip replacement operations than were allowed for under the funding formula, no additional funding would be provided. As with other public hospitals Warrnambool Base Hospital remains highly dependent on public funding for services provided, with ninety-three per cent of patients being public patients. Of the seven per cent classified as private patients, a proportion are funded by the Department of Veterans' Affairs or Workcover. Some privately insured patients, who receive treatment at the Hospital, do not use their private insurance because of the gap in the funding arrangements. Because of the quality of health care provided by Warrnambool Base Hospital to public patients there has been little incentive for most Warrnambool residents to take out private hospital cover. As a matter of policy, patients are admitted to the Hospital on the basis of need rather than whether or not they have private insurance cover. There is no distinction between public and private ward treatment, and patients at Warrnambool normally have access to a doctor of their choice. Although the board and management of the the Hospital was generally in favour of the introduction of casemix funding, they were obviously less enthusiastic about the former Coalition Government's reductions in funding for Victoria's public hospitals.

As the region's largest public hospital, Warrnambool Base was probably in a better position to respond to the introduction of the casemix management funding formula and cuts in government funding than smaller public hospitals in south-west Victoria. Several of these eventually succumbed to pressure to close or rationalise services, particularly acute care work. At the time of these reforms, in the early 1990s, the Kennett Government stated that a reduction in expenditure for Victoria's rural hospitals was justified in order to enable additional funding for Melbourne's outer suburban hospitals. The government argued that country hospitals were over-resourced, servicing only thirty-two per cent of the population while receiving thirty-five per cent of available State Government funding. It was also pointed out that while city public hospitals had long waiting lists this was not an issue for most country hospitals.

The reduction in State Government expenditure required the Hospital's senior management to make a careful assessment of the services provided. Given that this Hospital is assessed on the quality and number of medical services provided, the administration sought to identify and reduce non-essential services. As a result, though the ratio of nurses to beds was actually increased, the Hospital reduced the number of staff employed in nurse administration, in environmental services — which included cleaning and engineering — and in finance. The most striking example in the staff reductions was in catering, where staffing is now only half of what it was a decade ago. Staff cuts in the catering department were made possible by the introduction of new technology. A chill food system was introduced which enabled meals to be prepared in advance and meant that the Hospital did not need to employ weekend catering staff. In this instance staff cuts did not lead to industrial action and were achieved through attrition and voluntary redundancy packages. It was pointed out to the catering staff that the alternative to staff reductions was to privatise the catering service. The lack of industrial action is not surprising as Warrnambool is much less a union town than, say, Portland, Geelong or Bendigo. According to the current CEO, successful rationalisation of services helped to place Warrnambool Base Hospital in a sound financial situation by the end of the 1990s.

The introduction of the casemix funding for regional hospitals led to the closure of several smaller country hospitals such as Mortlake Community Hospital and pressure on others to work in a more complementary fashion with the major regional health providers such as Warrnambool Base Hospital.

It also changed the function of smaller public hospitals in south-west Victoria, which became less involved in acute care work.

Despite some staff reductions in the 1990s, Warrnambool Hospital remained the largest employer in the city. Of the Hospital's current budget of $46 million, seventy per cent is spent on salaries, with a high proportion of this remaining in Warrnambool. From an average staffing of approximately 700 a decade ago, in 1999 the Hospital employed 421 equivalent full time staff. This figure refers to staff employed on the Warrnambool campus of South West Health Care only and does not include staff employed in the privatised radiology and pathology departments. If staff employed by the Hospital outside of Warrnambool, particularly in the area of psychiatric services, are included, the total equivalent full time number of staff employed today is approximately 630. The value of the Hospital as the city's major employer of skilled, relatively highly paid labour, is underestimated by most residents of Warrnambool. While headlines in the *Standard* highlight job losses in the town's major manufacturing industries such as Fletcher Jones and Nestlé, far less publicity has been given to quite dramatic employment growth in the health and related aged care industries.

[1] *Standard*, Thursday 1 November 1984.

[2] *Standard*, 18 March, 1987.

[3] Warrnambool and District Base Hospital Annual Report (WDBH), 1986–87, Chairman's Report, p.6.

[4] WDBH Annual Report, 1988–89, p.15.

Chapter 18

MAJOR CHANGES AND EVENTS 1972–2000

Over a twenty-eight year period changing policy framework saw the Hospital evolve from being a general base hospital to being the key provider of health services for Victoria's south-western region. This chapter provides a brief outline of some of the more significant developments and events that occurred within the Hospital between 1972 and 2000 not covered thus far.

Compared to both the eighties and nineties, the 1970s was a decade of relative stability and steady growth for the Hospital. In 1972 a local dentist, Viv Balmer, was president of what was then the Hospital's committee of management with Alan Matthews the managing secretary. The organisational language used to describe the state public hospital system very much reflected its community-charitable origins. Alveston and Corio were still referred to in the Hospital's 1973–74 Annual Report as "Old Folks Homes" while a Hospital and Charities Commission had responsibility for administering Victoria's public hospitals on behalf of the State Government. Yet even in the early 1900s the Hospital was moving towards reducing the number of long term aged care inpatients.

V.G.C. Balmer, board president 1973–75

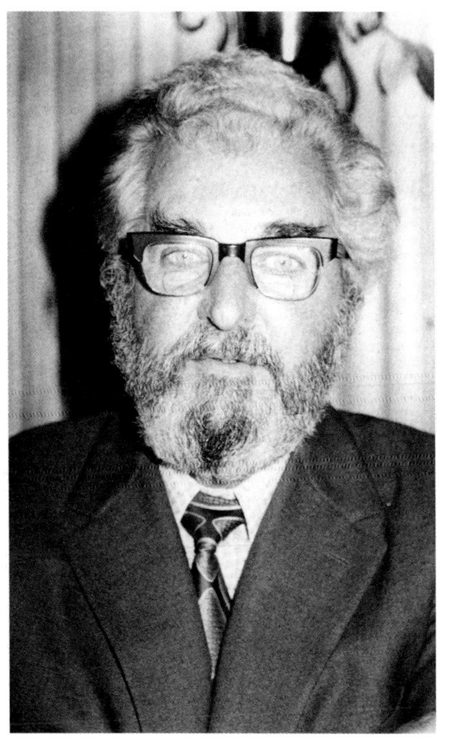

In announcing the appointment of a specialist geriatrician, Dr T. Howson, Mr Balmer in the President's report in 1974 noted the Committee had "accepted his philosophy" of "providing medical and paramedical services to support and maintain the elderly in their normal home environment with a view to delaying admission to a Nursing Home"[1]. Dr Howson had been appointed to the Hospital's recently established Geriatric Unit with plans to extend the Unit's services to the Warrnambool Shire.

In the early 1970s as well as applying for specific grants to the HCC, the Hospital still relied heavily on money raised from various auxiliaries to purchase equipment or undertake minor improvements to the buildings. During the year

1973–74 the local commercial radio station 3YB's Radio Appeal raised an all-time record sum of $80,527 for the Hospital. The various Ladies' Auxiliaries raised $12,549 while an Egg Appeal conducted by local schools contributed $436 to the Hospital's budget. Apart from financial assistance, volunteers from the local Warrnambool community contributed to the work of the Hospital through "constant rounds of visitations and other good works". In the 1973–74 annual report Mr Balmer noted how these "visitations" by volunteers "demonstrated compassion and thoughtfulness in an otherwise materialistic society".

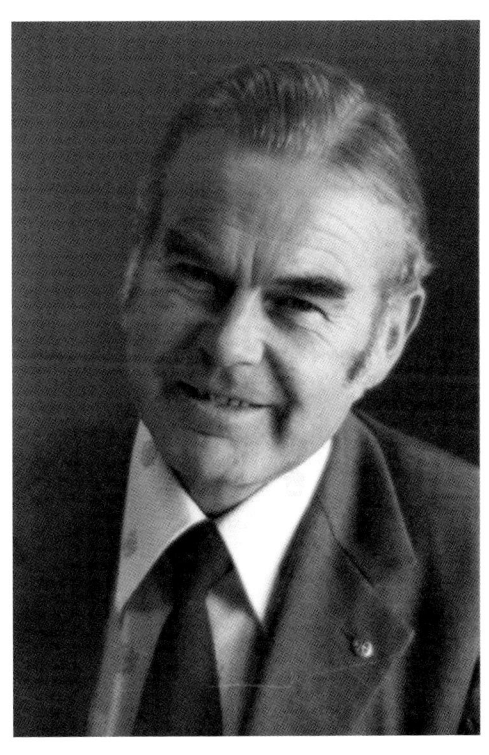

Alan Matthews, manager-secretary 1973–83

During the 1970s while the numbers of inpatients and outpatients increased steadily every year, the average length of stay per inpatient declined significantly. From 1971–72 to 1973–74 the number of inpatients treated increased from 5,175 to 5,889 while the average stay in hospital declined from 12.0 to 10.6 days. The numbers of outpatients increased quite dramatically with an attendance of 18,020 in 1971–72 rising to 28,289 in 1973–74.

In the early 1970s the Hospital had medical specialists only in the areas of geriatrics, radiology and pathology with the local GPs still very much involved in obstetrics, anaesthetics and general surgery. The medical superintendent, Dr John Reid, had overall responsibility for the care and treatment of patients while the matron, Miss June Stewart, exercised firm control over the nursing staff which comprised young single women living in the Hospital's nurses home.

By far the most significant policy change that affected the Hospital in the 1970s was the Federal Labor Government's Medibank programme in July 1975. According to the Chairman of the Hospital's Committee of Management in 1975 the introduction of Medibank was for Victoria's public hospitals "a quite revolutionary change in the procedure and philosophy associated with the delivery of health care services to communities"[2]. The introduction of Medibank by the Federal Labor Government brought to an end the appointment of visiting medical specialists who had formerly provided treatment on honorary basis for patients unable to pay.

The Victorian State Government also took increased responsibility for the funding, hence operation, of the state's public hospitals. As part of the implementation of the Syme Townsend Report into the future administration of Victoria's public hospital system, from 1975 the management of the Base Hospital had to deal with the newly established Victorian Health Services Commission. Victoria's public hospitals, which had been largely autonomous, community-based institutions, were now increasingly part of an integrated state and regional health system.

In August 1976 Dr John Reid, who had worked at the Hospital for seventeen years, at first as a pathologist then as a medical superintendent, retired. In the 1976–77 Annual Report his successor, Dr P.G. Morton, referred to Dr Reid's departure as a "sombre occasion for the medical fraternity". In his detailed report Dr Morton makes several interesting observations. After commenting on the "inadequate number of general practitioners in country areas", Dr Morton referred to "pressure brought to bear on the future to . . . restrict the access of general practitioners to patients in hospitals". Referring to recent moves on the part of the Victorian State Government to exert greater control over the operation of the state's public hospitals, Dr Morton noted "The role of the Hospital has to be redefined. Hospitals are no longer isolated institutions on the Hill; they are part of overall Health Services"[3].

In his 1976 report as Medical Superintendent Dr Morton makes yet another reference to "the calibre of doctors" engaged at the Hospital, who provide "expertise in all fields necessary for a community of this size". According to Dr Morton during the "Medibank upheaval" in 1975 — with many doctors strongly opposed to the scheme — "no patient suffered a lack of medical care through any industrial action . . . a far different situation from many other places in Australia"[4].

Apart from the introduction of Medibank the other major policy reform that the Hospital's Committee of Management had to grapple with was the State Government's regionalisation of health services. What had been largely autonomously managed public hospitals were increasingly to become subject to the State Government policies implemented by the Health Commission — later the Department of Health and Community Services. As with other State Government bureaucracies, the funding, hence policy directions, of publicly funded health services including base hospitals was to become part of a regional health service. In his 1977–78 report as president of the Hospital's board of management, Mr E. Johnson refers to the "advent of the new Health Commission which has given rise to much conjecture and debate on the question of expanding the regional concept of delivering health services throughout Victoria"[5].

The medical superintendent, Dr P.G. Morton's report dated 16 August 1978, provides a detailed description of the range of medical and health related services provided by the Hospital at the end of the 1970s. In his report Dr Morton notes the arrival and departure of medical staff including a reference to a "young, enthusiastic and highly qualified" Dr Sean Rogan from Ireland who "had settled well into the medical and social life in Warrnambool". Two young pharmacists, Miss Christine Lightfoot and Mr Allan Luke had also been recruited from the United Kingdom which enabled the pharmacy department to "further its involvement in pre-natal nutrition, intravenous additives and regional pharmacy"[6]. The Hospital's pharmacy now also met the drug requirements of the "Timboon, Koroit, Terang, Camperdown and Port Fairy" district hospitals.

Dr Morton's report, in providing details of the increased role of the Hospital's welfare department which referred people to district nursing and home help and the Day Hospital, alludes to three of the major changes which were to be of increasing significance during the 1980s. These were the recruitment of specialist medical staff from overseas, the Hospital's growing role as a regional health care provider and the expansion of community based health care.

By far the most dramatic event in the early 1980s in both Warrnambool and the Hospital's history was the tragedy of the Ash Wednesday (16 February 1983) bushfires which resulted in seven deaths as well as heavy stock losses. During this period the Hospital treated forty-four casualties only one of whom needed to be transferred to the Royal Melbourne Hospital for treatment. The seven bodies of those who died were brought to the Hospital.

The treatment of fire victims was made more difficult by a two-hour blackout when SEC powerlines were destroyed. There was an obvious need for the Hospital to upgrade its emergency power supply and successfully applied to the State Government for $300,000 to purchase a new generator. The year 1983 also saw a major upgrading of the rehabilitation unit, Ward 9 and the return of the physiotherapy unit to the main hospital site from premises in Timor Street. Two important changes in senior personnel occurred during 1983 with Peter McGregor commencing as CEO in August and Dr Glynne Priddle replacing Dr John Callaghan as director of medical services in November.

In February 1984 the Federal Labor Government introduced Medicare as part of its universal health care policy, which had implications for the Hospital's funding and mix of patients. During 1984 the number of public patients admitted to the Hospital increased by thirty-eight per cent. The Hospital responded by reducing the cost of a private, single bed ward from $180 to $130 per day. In terms of state government policy, 1984 saw the regionalisation of health service become a reality with the appointment of John McLelland as Director of the Barwon Regional Health Service, which included Warrnambool. In 1984 the work of the Hospital was still supported by a number of auxiliaries which included a Senior and Junior Ladies Auxiliary and Community Auxiliaries at Nullawarre/Mepunga, Nirranda and Woolsthorpe. The Caramut Ladies Auxiliary had closed in 1983.

As part of the general broadening of services the Hospital started a weekly family planning clinic in April 1984 with funding and staff provided by the Health Commission. The 1984–85 annual report referred to the previous twelve months as a "Year of industrial turmoil with the Hospital needing to use volunteers on occasions to keep the Hospital functioning"[7].

During the early and mid 1980s the Hospital continued to experience difficulties in attracting and retaining qualified nursing staff. The 1984–85 Annual Report also referred to the staged transfer of nurse training to a college based course with a Diploma in Nursing to commence at Warrnambool Institute in 1986.

The year 1985 saw a number of new senior appointments with Dr Ian Carsons commencing as director of medical services in September, Dr Darra Murphy appointed as his deputy director and director of emergency services and Miss Lois Lindsay to replace Miss Jean Edgar as director of nursing. The 1984–85 report also noted the recent resignation of the Hospital's audiologist, George Lancaster and the appointment of Bore Hoekstra as chief physiotherapist and Ruth Heller as coordinator of the recently established Sexual Assault Unit (now Centre for Sexual Assault).

The process of regionalising Victoria's health services continued with the establishment of various working groups to work with the newly appointed regional director, Tony Ryan, made up of hospital board presidents, CEOs, directors of nursing and nurse educators. During the mid-1980s to late 1980s Warrnambool Base Hospital continued to treat increasing members of shorter term patients. The 1986–87 Annual Report noted that the number of inpatients had increased by 755 or 12.36% though the total number of patient days had actually decreased from 50,970 to 47,160 due to a reduction in the average length of stay from 8.2 to 6.8 days[8].

Of major concern to the Hospital management over the late 1980s was how to achieve the Hospital's performance target given the cuts in state government funding. These not only impacted on the Hospital's annual operating costs but also, in February 1988, led to a modification of the Rehabilitation Unit's redevelopment following a cut in funding from $6.5 million to $4 million. Another major, potentially sensitive, area of concern at this time for the Hospital administration was the number of nursing home type patients who were occupying beds needed for acute care patients.

During the mid-1980s to late 1980s the number of surgical cases increased steadily, in part reflecting the improved facilities and increased number of surgeons working at the Hospital. The 1989–90 Annual Report contains initial reference to the construction of a new, larger and improved operating suite as part of a $5.6 million redevelopment[9].

Most of the major changes which the Hospital responded to during the 1980s continued during the 1990s. During the 1990s virtually every one of the Hospital's annual reports contains details of new health services provided or facilitated by the Hospital. For example the 1992–93 Annual Report refers to the establishment of a Continence Management Clinic, a Diabetes Education Resource Unit and the development of critical care and stomal therapy in palliative care units[10]. By the mid-1990s Warrnambool Base Hospital had become a sophisticated and comprehensive public hospital with fewer patients needing to be transferred to Melbourne for treatment.

Throughout the 1990s, in spite of reductions in state government funding,

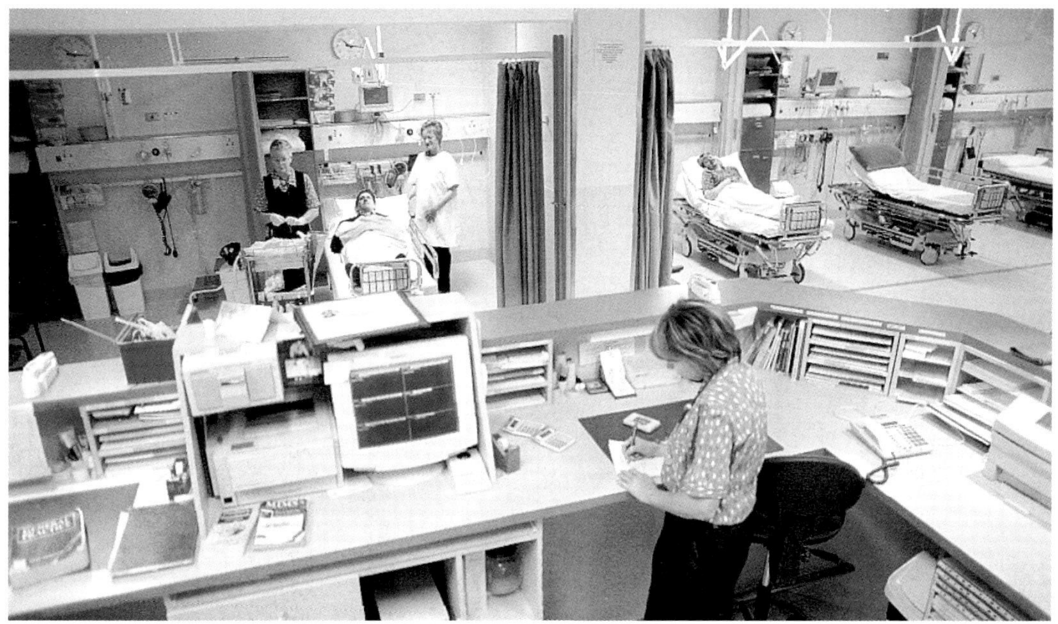

New Emergency Department 1999

the Hospital continued to purchase expensive medical equipment and undertake major extensions and refurbishments of its buildings. In September 1993 an official ceremony was held to mark the opening of a new allied health building and medical records building together with the reopening of the rehabilitation ward, which had been closed for twenty months. The new operating theatre and emergency department facilities were opened in June 1998 which the Hospital's 1997–98 annual report claimed "reinforces and consolidates the Hospital as the major sub-referral centre for the south-west region"[11]. This report also notes the relocation of the Hospital's health and information services to the former emergency department which provided increased office space for medical records and which integrated health information services and the emergency reception and inpatients admission into one area. In 1998 Hider Street was closed to traffic which divided the Hospital's recently constructed Acute Psychotic Unit from the main site.

[1] WDBH 120 Annual Report, 1973–74.
[2] WDBH 122 Annual Report, 1975–76, p.4.
[3] WDBH Annual Report 1975–76, p.14.
[4] WDBH Annual Report, 1975–76, p.11.
[5] WDBH Annual Report, 1977–78.
[6] WDBH Annual Report, 1977–78, p.10.
[7] WDBH Annual Report, 1984–85, p.2
[8] WDBH Annual Report, 1986–87, p.5
[9] WDBH Annual Report, 1989–90.
[10] WDBH Annual Report, 1992–93.
[11] WDBH 1997-98 Annual Report, p.2.

Chapter 19

DOCTORS AND NURSES 1972–2000

Between 1972 and 2000 the Hospital changed from a community hospital into a key provider of acute and related health care for its region. The number, professional background and conditions of employment of medical practitioners and nursing staff changed to meet the need to provide more specialised, acute care services in a more exacting regulatory and legal framework.The Hospital increasingly needed to employ well-qualified health professionals. During the past two decades Warrnambool's development as one of Victoria's key regional hospitals has been largely due to the management's success in attracting and retaining vital medical, nursing and allied health professional staff. Recruitment and retention of highly qualified staff have been and remain one of the major challenges facing Victoria's rural hospitals. Major changes in the state government's health policies during the 1980s and 1990s had the potential to generate major disputes between management and the Hospital's medical and nursing staff. Due in part to the Hospital's sound financial position and a flexible response on the part of management to potentially divisive issues such as negotiation of work contracts with doctors, industrial disputes between management and the medical staff have been rare.

Over the past two decades increase in patient demand for specialist medical services, especially in the areas of obstetrics and general surgery, together with changes in the regulatory and legal framework in which medicine is practised in Australia, has seen specialists largely replace GPs in larger public and private hospitals. Although some GPs resented being excluded from performing deliveries or general surgery at the Hospital, the majority have continued to enjoy a good working relationship with both the management and medical specialists. For most local GPs it was not so much a matter of being pushed out of the Hospital by specialists, but more their own choice to exclude themselves.

This situation has changed a great deal since 1975 when according to Dr Harry Savery, who arrived in Warrnambool from England that year "the GPs largely ran the Hospital". Dr Savery's decision to cease medical practice in the United Kingdom was in part due to the extent to which GPs in Britain were being excluded from working in hospitals in favour of specialists. At the Warrnambool Base Hospital Dr Savery was pleased to find local GPs regularly "met with and learnt greatly from consultants . . . who

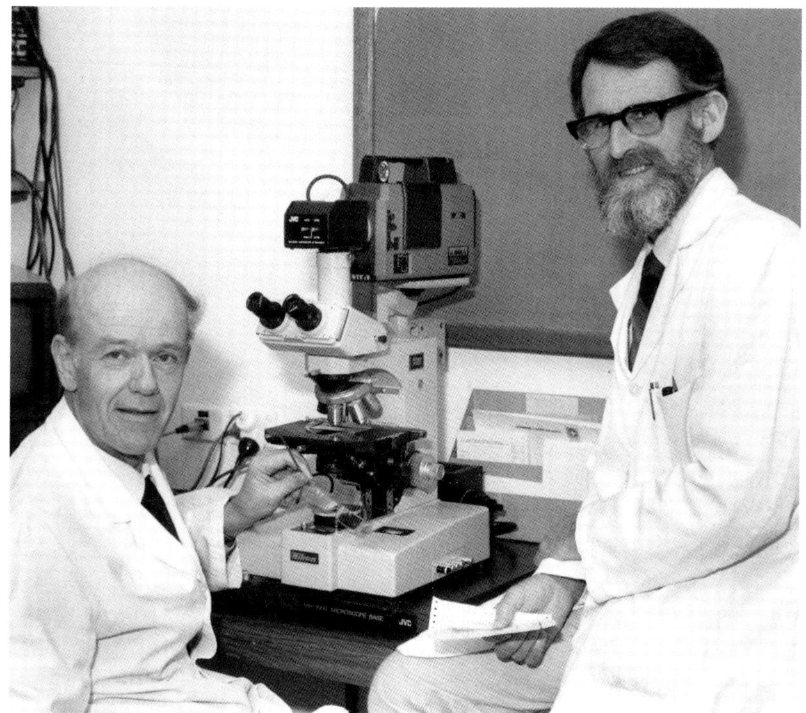

Pathologist Dr Eric Pihl (left), and laboratory manager Geoff O'Brien, with the pathology department's video equipped microscope.

enjoyed a mutually beneficial relationship and ultimately the patients benefited". Commenting on the situation in the late 1990s, Dr Savery observed that though local "GPs had been displaced at the Hospital . . . a good working relationship existed between the two groups with [a] clinical meeting every week". Based on his experiences as a GP in Warrnambool for almost a quarter of a century, Dr Savery formed a view that "specialists in country hospitals are very approachable . . . with interchange between specialists and GPs . . . much better than in the city". Clearly this level of cooperation between local medical practitioners who generally socialise as well as work together is one of the strengths of the Warrnambool Base Hospital.

In the south-west region, there has been an increased centralisation of medical practitioners in Warrnambool, as a growing service centre for an expanding catchment area. Having achieved a critical mass of well-qualified medical practitioners by the late 1980s it has become easier for the Hospital to attract and retain both recently graduated doctors and medical specialists. This was certainly not the case in January 1986 when a shortage of resident medical officers (RMOs) forced the Hospital to close the Outpatients Department for several weeks. This was at a time when a general shortage of doctors was affecting the operation of most of Victoria's country hospitals. At the beginning of 1986 the Hospital had only been able to recruit two RMOs rather than the six needed to staff the Hospital including the Outpatients Department[1]. This problem had arisen due to Melbourne's metropolitan hospitals taking more interns rather than any reduction in the number of medical graduates. According to the executive director of the Victorian branch of the AMA, many graduates took internships in Melbourne in order to undertake specialist training. At one stage the Hospital's director of medical services, Dr Ian Carson proposed "sponsoring a doctor from overseas after all attempts to fill all vacancies had failed"[2]. One option rejected by Dr Carson at the time was to request the RMOs to work longer hours as these doctors were already on duty for over a hundred hours per week. In 1988, when the Hospital still faced a shortage of RMOs, having been able to fill only three out of five positions, consideration was given to recruiting from Ireland or the United Kingdom.

Faced with the difficulty of attracting specialists to Warrnambool during the 1980s the Hospital board successfully recruited a number of specialists from overseas. In September 1986, Dr Carson, stated in the Hospital's Annual Report that the expansion of specialist services was "perhaps the most exciting event of the year".[3] The *Standard* announced "the imminent arrival of Mr Brendan Mooney, a specialist urologist from Limerick, Ireland, who accepted a position of surgeon specialising in urinary system and kidneys". Mr Mooney's wife, Dr Claire Mooney, who commenced general practice in Warrnambool, also held an appointment at the Hospital. Another key appointment was that of a Mr Lukas Hartanto, the regional specialist geriatrician who had previously been employed in a teaching hospital in Sweden. In the same year, the Hospital also recruited two specialist pathologists (Dr Mike Robson and Dr David Blaxland) and a specialist anaesthetist (Dr Jim Barson) while Dr Mark Ivers from Melbourne joined as a specialist psychiatrist. In the Hospital's 1988 Annual Report Dr Carson stated that "during the past twelve months (the Hospital) has been able to add to its staff a second consultant paediatrician, a full time drug and alcohol position, a consultant orthopaedic surgeon, a visiting oral surgeon and a visiting oncology service with two consultants".[4] These additional appointments promoted the Board's aspirations for the Hospital to become a truly sub-regional referral centre with a broad range of specialist medical services.

Dr George Awburn and Mrs Awburn with Stewart Lindsay at his retirement dinner, June 1972.

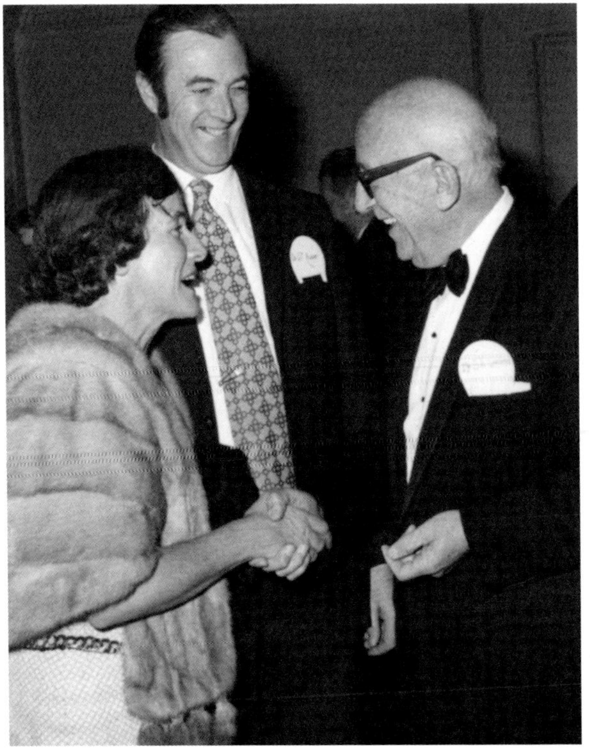

The appointment of additional specialists in the mid-1980s meant decreasing opportunities for local GPs to work at the Hospital. Several responded by developing their own areas of specialisation. For example in 1984 Dr Eric Fairbank, who had arrived in Warrnambool in 1974, was a key member of a committee to establish a palliative care programme within the Hospital. The Palliative Care Unit, one of the first in Victoria outside Melbourne, was established at the Hospital in 1986.

The management of the Hospital showed similar flexibility in encouraging another local GP, Dr Roger Brough, to develop expertise in the area of drug and alcohol rehabilitation. After completing two years as an RMO at the Hospital, Dr Brough was offered a partnership by Dr George Awburn in his general practice. Dr Brough was subsequently involved in the Hospital's drink driver programme and a local venture to sell non-alcoholic drinks in Warrnambool. During the late 1970s Dr Brough was a member of a steering committee to establish the Warrnambool Association of Alcohol and Drug Dependence (WRAAD) which in 1986 became the Warrnambool and Western Region's Alcohol and Drug Centre (WRAD). In 1984 Dr Brough spent six months in Melbourne to undertake a work and study programme in drug and alcohol dependence. Following his return to Warrnambool Dr Brough was offered a new position with the Hospital as a drug and alcohol specialist. In creating this position the Hospital was following the NSW model which places greater emphasis on a medical approach to drug and alcohol related treatment than the community-based approach more typical of Victoria. In both these instances the Hospital management had the financial capacity and flexibility to enable two capable and enthusiastic local GPs to develop much needed areas of specialist expertise.

Some of Warrnambool's older GPs experienced considerable difficulty in adjusting to decreased opportunities to work at the Hospital. Reflecting on his decision to purchase a solo practice in Warrnambool in 1958, one of Warrnambool's longest serving GPs, Dr Les Hemingway, stated in 1997 "Now I wouldn't come here . . . I'd go to Colac or somewhere else like that where they [GPs] haven't been pushed out by specialists". In the 1990s Dr Hemingway was particularly angry when a recently arrived specialist anaesthetist refused to give anaesthetics for local GPs who had previously performed general surgery at the Hospital. According to Dr Hemingway, this particular anaesthetist failed to take into account the impressive track record of Warrnambool's GPs in performing general surgery often under extremely difficult circumstances when no specialist surgeon was available. Since the arrival of two specialist obstetricians in Warrnambool in the early 1980s Dr Hemingway and most other local GPs had decreasing opportunities to deliver babies at the Hospital. The high cost of litigation insurance was also a factor in explaining why most local GPs moved out of obstetrics. Dr Hemingway who "used to do over a hundred (deliveries) a year" in 1958–59, reported that by 1997 "it had got down to one a year".

The reasons stated by medical specialists for accepting positions at the

Hospital are interesting and varied. One factor common to all was their perception of Warrnambool as an attractive coastal centre with excellent facilities and within a reasonable distance of Melbourne. As well as providing them and their families with an enviable lifestyle, the Hospital provided doctors with a congenial and professionally stimulating working environment.

In this regard, the observations of Dr Nick Thies, who first came to Warrnambool as a fifth year medical student and returned initially as a first year RMO in 1972 and subsequently as a specialist paediatrician, are worth quoting in detail. Explaining his subsequent decision to establish himself as a paediatrician in Warrnambool, Dr Thies states:

> I went to England for two years and then to Queen Victoria Hospital in Melbourne for one year and then to the Royal Children's Hospital for three years. During this time I was training as a paediatrician and also, whilst I was in Melbourne, I travelled down to Warrnambool for holidays as I had a basic ambition to return to Warrnambool as I enjoyed the lifestyle. I also wanted to get to know the GPs and get a feel for whether a paediatrician was needed. At this time there was no fully trained paediatrician.
>
> So in 1980 I set up on my own as a paediatrician (in Warrnambool). The first eight years were very hectic — it was a twenty-four hour a day job, every day, as I was the only paediatrician and it did not take me very long to build up my practice. Most GPs had to deal with paediatrics before I came but they were uncomfortable about this and they liked being able to refer a child locally without having to send them on long distances. In 1988 Peter Forrest came and set up with me and that made a huge difference. It meant I only had to work every second weekend and I had every second night off without being on call. I could take more holidays without feeling guilty. Before then if I went away for a few days I would feel guilty as I approached Warrnambool worrying about how many sick kids were waiting for me. I'd go straight down to the Hospital, often without even unpacking. If someone got sick before I was due to go away for a weekend I would have to stay.
>
> What I particularly liked about setting up in Warrnambool was that I could set it up and work my own waY . . . I also enjoyed the camaraderie of all the doctors in town, it was really very good. Every morning after the ward rounds we would have morning tea together. We would yarn and have a medical talk or sandwiches and bikkies. But now no one has the time for that — everyone tends to be too busy.

Dr Thies's comments on the working atmosphere of the Warrnambool Base Hospital compared to British and Melbourne training hospitals are also revealing.

> When I first came to Warrnambool I liked the idea that everyone knew each other in the different departments whether in the medical team or the engineers or the administrators or the caterers or cleaners — there was no snobbery. When I was a student I took a job in St Andrews doing repair jobs like changing light globes etc. and the snobbery there really got up

> my nose. I was dressed in overalls in the elevator one day and said "hello" to the consultant in the lift with me and he put his nose up in the air and completely ignored me. None of that snobbery exists down here. In Melbourne in the med world you get the feeling that you have got to know where your place is and don't climb too high. In England I went to see a consultant who walked along with the registrar and house physicians behind him. He was very much on his high horse — to work with him was deemed by him to be a privilege; I chose not to work with him.

Dr Thies notes how Warrnambool's GPs and medical specialists have been able to "overcome the isolation of working in rural areas". Dr Thies belongs "to a television journal club —

> Every six weeks twenty to thirty paediatricians all get on the phone together — three present journal articles. There is also another group that have teleconferences and invite a speaker to speak to them for about half an hour and there are questions and discussions. There are regular updates at the Children's Hospital and an annual conference on one topic and then a postgraduate forum of overseas and Australian speakers which is open to all paediatricians. Another group get together for a conference over the long weekend or three to four days with wives. We also have a Satellite Clinic where a geneticist comes to Warrnambool twice a year to give a clinic at the Hospital. Bookings are made through the Children's Hospital.

In terms of the growth and more specialised nature of the Hospital's medical workforce it is interesting to compare the Hospital's honorary and departmental medical officers listed in the 1973–74 Annual Report with their equivalents whose details are included in the Hospital's 1997–98 Annual Report. In the twenty-four year period the number of qualified medical and dental officers from forty-three to eighty-seven. While the number of departmental (or employed) medical officers was seven in both 1974 and 1998, the number of visiting medical and dental officers increased from thirty-six to seventy-nine. During this period the population of the City of Warrnambool increased by approximately one third — from around 19,000 to 30,000. Hence the increase in the Hospital's medical and dental establishment was largely due to a steady increase in the demand for acute care medical services within the south-west region. Many patients within a radius of up to 150 kilometres of Warrnambool, who formerly needed to go to Geelong, Ballarat or Melbourne for specialised medical treatment, are now treated by doctors in Warrnambool.

The growth of specialist medical services available at the Hospital is apparent if one compares the number and range of medical specialists associated with the Hospital in 1974 and 1998[5]. In providing details of honorary medical officers the 1973–74 annual report lists two general surgeons (Mr J.W. Fisher and Mr A. Fligelman), two specialist obstetricians (as opposed to GPs with qualifications in obstetrics) Dr J. Brookes and Dr I.P. Scott[6] (who is also listed as a paediatrician) and a specialist ophthalmologist (Dr G. Jones). The same report does not provide details of any

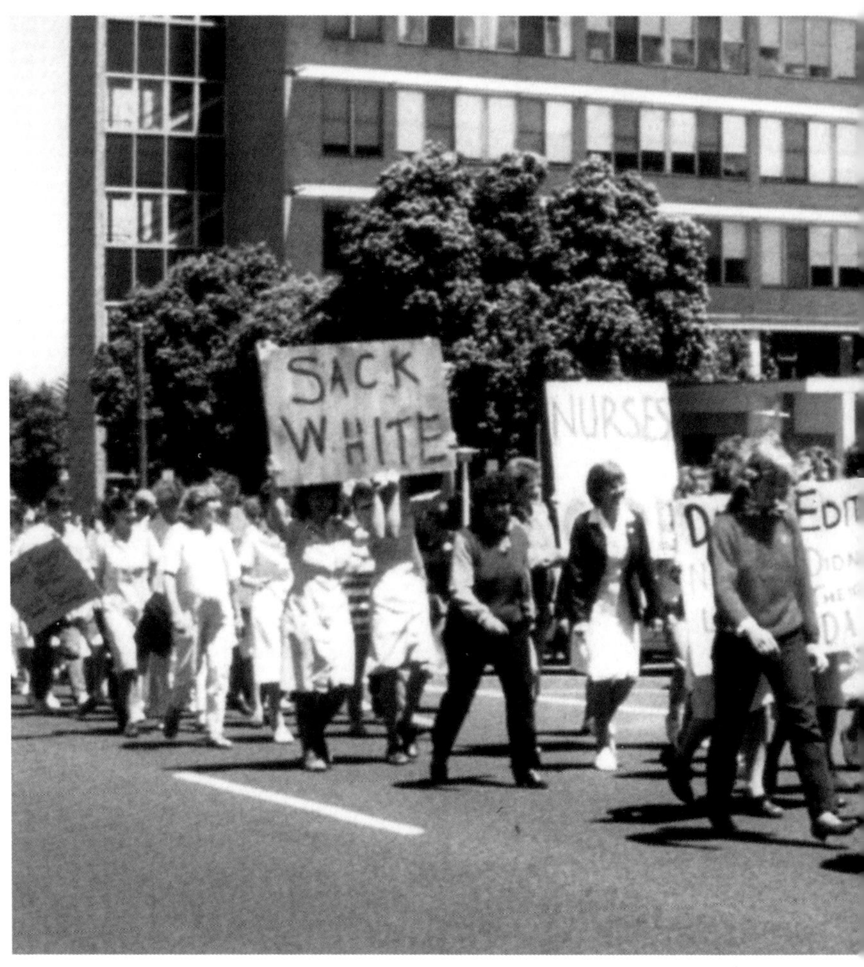

specialist anaesthetists or radiologists. By way of contrast the Hospital's 1997–98 Annual Report lists six specialist anaesthetists (Drs P. Arnold, P. Cronin, A. Dawson, G. Kilminister, G. Mullins and K. Prest) and nine radiologists (Drs D. Boldt, M. Bennett, A. McLaughlan, E. Phelan, J.M. Rogan, A. Slaven, P. Tauro, P. Walker and R. White). By 1998 the Hospital's medical specialists also included two orthopaedic surgeons (Mr M. Dooley and Mr N.A. Sundaram) three obstetricians and gynaecologists (Dr C. Beaton, Dr K. Braniff and Dr I. Pettigrew) two paediatricians (Dr G. Pallas and Dr N. Thies) and a renal physician (Dr R. Auwardt). In 1974 the Hospital's "departmental (employed) officers" simply consisted of a medical superintendent (Dr John Reid) and six RMOs including the well-known Warrnambool doctors Dr John Philpot, Dr Roger Brough and the late Dr Eric Maxwell. In 1998 as well as a director (Dr P. O'Brien) and deputy director of medical services (Dr D.S. Pedler) the Hospital departmental officers included a director of anaesthetics (Dr K. Prest), a director of critical care unit (Dr B. Morphett) and a director of palliative care (Dr E. Fairbank).

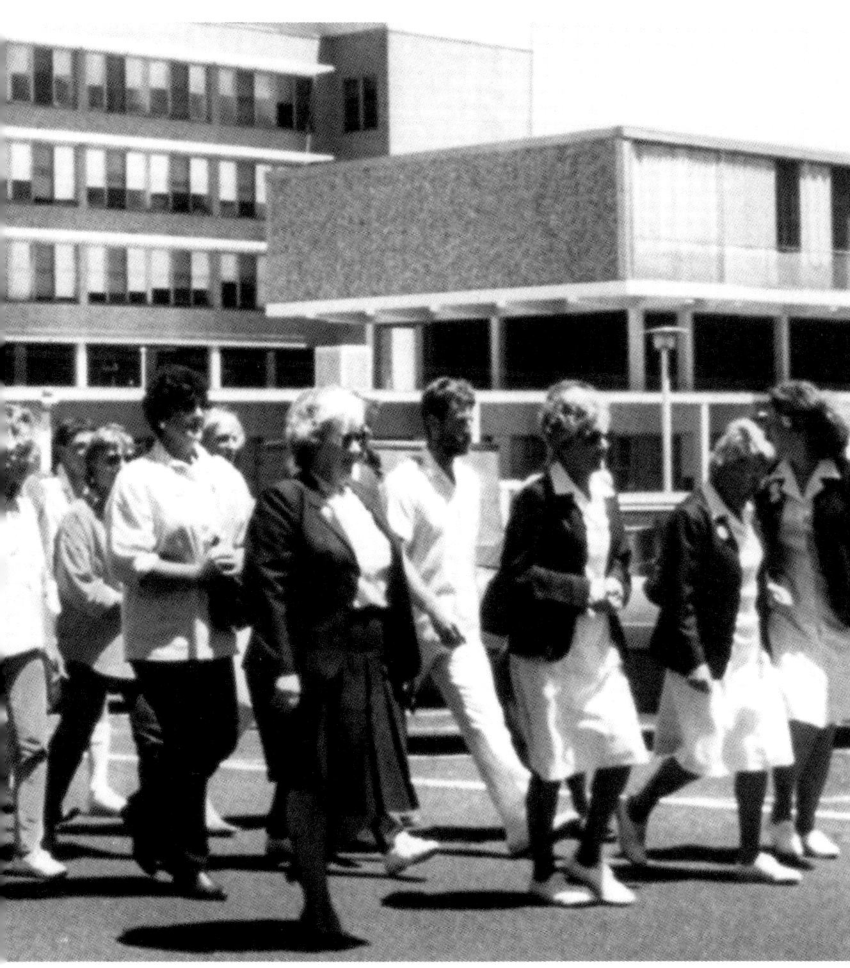

Nurses march past the Hospital, during the 1986 nursing dispute.

NURSES

In Chapter 14, it was suggested that while great changes took place in the buildings and quality of patient care at Warrnambool Base Hospital during the 1945–72 period, the training, work and conditions of employment of nurses remained essentially the same. This has certainly not been true of the last quarter of the twentieth century. As is the case in other Australian hospitals, the registered nursing staff employed at South West Healthcare today have little in common with their predecessors in 1972, most of whom were single female trainees who were still required to undertake a great deal of unskilled, non-nursing duties. As was the case with senior staff of private girls' schools, positions of responsibility in nursing were the preserve of unmarried career sisters who lived on the premises and generally had reputations as stern disciplinarians.

As in the other caring professions, the last two decades of this century have seen quite fundamental changes in the recruitment, education, work, conditions of employment, marital and professional status and sex of nurses. For the most part, education and conditions of employment at Warrnambool Base Hospital since 1972 reflect developments in the profession within Australia and most western countries. These developments also reflect changes in the traditional role of women in western societies. While nurses employed in Australian regional hospitals have similar work and conditions of employment to nurses employed in large metropolitan hospitals, there are some significant differences. According to Sue Morrison, the current director of nursing, though a growing proportion of nurses employed at the Hospital have undertaken a university course in nursing and are then recruited from outside the region, most are locals. Unlike their colleagues working in large metropolitan hospitals, nurses employed at regional hospitals like Warrnambool, normally live, shop and socialise in the local community that the Hospital serves. Given their situation, it would seem reasonable to assume that nurses employed in regional hospitals have a better understanding of patients' backgrounds and their local community than their metropolitan counterparts.

Ms Morrison was first employed as a trainee nurse in 1968. She recalls that her duties then were "more task orientated" and included "squeezing oranges for juice, doing the flowers and dusting the lockers". By the late 1970s, it was apparent that the Hospital could no longer afford to use even trainee nurses to perform less skilled non-nursing work. This was partly due to a general shortage of nursing staff and an increasing number of acute care patients who for legal and medical reasons, required specialised nursing.

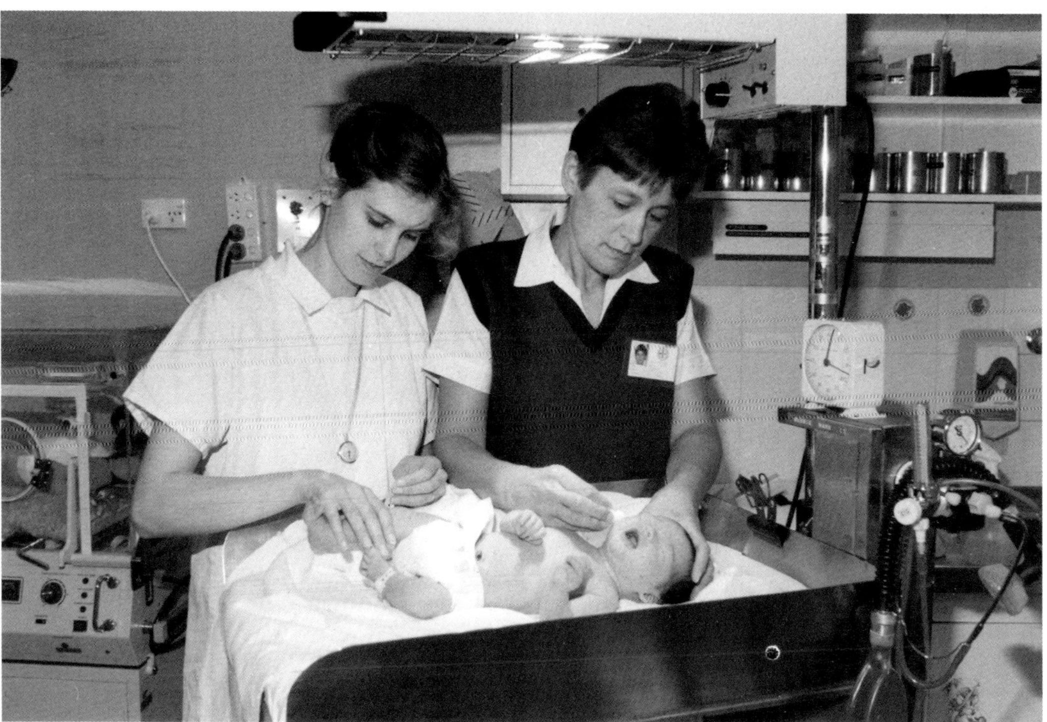

Midwifery staff Janet Hynes and Phyllis Walsh, at an open infant care cot, 1989.

An improvement in the professional standing of nurses, reflected in improved salaries and award conditions, was also an important consideration in explaining changes in the work and working conditions of nurses. As a consequence from the late 1970s on, the Hospital increasingly employed more general staff — cleaners, cooks and wardsmen — as well as making use of voluntary labour to perform non-nursing tasks. Since the mid-1980s university nursing trainees, completing required periods of supervised clinical practice, no longer provide the Hospital with a cheap source of labour as part of the requirements of training.

As with other Australian hospitals, increases in the acute care patient caseload required the Hospital not only to employ qualified, registered nurses, but to encourage them to undertake further specialised training. Initially the Hospital's decision to employ general staff to perform non-nursing duties resulted in a decrease in the number of nurses employed. According to Sue Morrison, with "fewer nurses being needed, at first . . . it went from seven on the ward, down to five in the morning and from five to four nurses in the afternoon". The Hospital's need for qualified, experienced nurses together with changes in society and legislation regarding employment opportunities for women has resulted in hospitals employing more married women as nurses. The employment of more mature, married women and men as nurses, together with the transfer of initial nurse training from hospitals to universities and TAFE Colleges, has had an obvious impact on the working conditions and work environment of nurses. Simply put, by the 1980s, the working conditions of nurses, which in certain respects were not dissimilar to those of a military camp or convent, had to change significantly if capable young people were to be attracted and retained in the profession. The hierarchical structure and culture of nursing, with nurses referred to by surname only, has been substantially modified to take account of changes in the educational and cultural background of the nursing workforce.

During the 1970s the training and the conditions of work of nurses employed at the Hospital remained basically unchanged. However during the 1980s nursing in Australia made significant moves towards gaining professional status with tertiary institutions, first colleges of advanced education, then universities, assuming the responsibility for formal education of registered nurses. The training of state enrolled nurses, whose numbers have steadily declined basically due to the legal requirements regarding the duties of nurses employed in hospitals, is now undertaken by the technical and further education sector (TAFE). The other major change in the employment of nurses in both metropolitan and regional hospitals has been the increased proportion employed in part time positions. At the Hospital these changes have basically reflected statewide and national trends.

In the early 1970s the great majority of young women selected as nursing trainees at the Hospital were from Warrnambool and the surrounding district. These young women, who were required to live in the nursing home, were closely supervised and wore uniforms that clearly designated their employment status at the Hospital. As trainee nurses, they undertook a great deal of work that would now be done by nursing aides and basically learned through on the job experience or completing short non-credit courses run by the Hospital. Most had relatively short careers as nurses as there was little provision for part time work after they had married. By the early 1980s the board and senior staff at the Hospital, as elsewhere, were aware of the need for trainee nurses to complete a formal tertiary qualification. According to Sue Morrison, nurses at Warrnambool first became aware of the availability of tertiary level courses in nursing through attending conferences and by reading the popular American journal *Nursing* which was available in the nurses' common room. By the mid-1980s it was inevitable that nurse education would move from a hospital-based nurse training programme to a tertiary-based training programme. Underlying this change was the nursing profession's and union's desire to enhance nursing's professional standing by requiring future nurses to hold recognised tertiary qualifications. There were concerns that hospital-based training was expensive and had limited capacity to provide trainee nurses with the more detailed scientific and technical knowledge required for acute care nursing.

In Warrnambool, the obvious solution was the development of a Diploma of Nursing course at the Warrnambool Institute of Advanced Education (WIAE), now Deakin University's Warrnambool campus. [7] However, following the publication of a report by the Victorian Post-Secondary Education Commission, it appeared that no nursing education course would be conducted in the south-west. The report, published in September 1984, recommended against the establishment of a college-based nurse training course at Warrnambool Institute and that the Hospital's current course be transferred to Deakin University, Geelong. One of the Commission's reasons for recommending "a tertiary educational nursing programme . . . at Geelong rather than Warrnambool" was that it felt "unable to recommend a course at Warrnambool . . . until the development at Deakin University in relationship with Geelong Hospital [was] known"[8]. In any event the Institute Council's and Hospital Board's joint representation to Commission and the State Government saw this recommendation ignored with a nurse education course commencing at WIAE in 1986. As with Australia's other non-metropolitan colleges of advanced education, the Institute in 1985 was keen to develop a nurse training programme which would create another faculty and attract students additional and Federal Government funding. In 1985 Tony Barnett was appointed foundation dean of nursing at WIAE, and the Institute enrolled its first intake of trainee nurses in the same year.

As one would expect, the Hospital's senior staff and board members had certain reservations regarding the transfer of the Hospital-based nurse training to tertiary institutions. Apart from the loss of the nurse trainee workforce, there was concern that the graduates of WIAE's Diploma of Nursing programme would lack the clinical expertise of nurses who had trained at the Hospital. To address these concerns, senior hospital staff and local medicos were involved in the development of course units.In the manner of student teachers, nursing students at WIAE were required to satisfactorily complete block periods of clinical practice in hospitals, including Warrnambool, within the region.

Over time, the initial problems and tensions between the Hospital and WIAE/Deakin regarding the pre-service training of nurses have been resolved. Pat Nesbitt, a nurse educator at Deakin since 1986, suggests that "the Hospital is part of the educational process and what has helped . . . is that now a lot of the present nurses have a tertiary background. They know what it is like trying to assimilate into a hospital and [are] much more sympathetic to some of the difficulties that new graduates are going to face".

In many instances the tertiary background of nurses at the Hospital extends well beyond the completion of a Bachelor of Nursing. At Warrnambool and elsewhere, it is now common practice for nurses to complete further specialist university courses, especially if they aspire to positions in management, such as masters programmes in health administration.

Deakin University proposals designed to promote collaborative research initiatives mainly in regional and rural health between the Hospitals and the University have been only partly successful. In the 1990s Deakin's School of Nursing sought to establish more formal links with the Hospital following the appointment of a Professor of Nursing at Warrnambool. One proposal involved the establishment of a professional unit within the Hospital to facilitate the development of collaborative research projects. The intention was for the professional position to span both institutions' management structures. According to Pat Nesbitt, this proposal "met with a brick wall with the former director of nursing who wasn't very supportive of establishing more formal links with Deakin". The possibility of establishing the professional unit, "which also would have allowed the University to learn a great deal more in the clinical area" was lost when the Professor of Nursing, Dirk Kayser, resigned and was not replaced. The current Director of Nursing, Sue Morrison, refers to other tensions between the two institutions in the mid-1990s relating to Hospital employment of Deakin nursing graduates. The Hospital apparently felt some pressure to employ local graduates who were overall less well qualified academically than applicants from other universities. For a brief period, Deakin nursing graduates were given bonus points to justify their appointment to the Hospital's staff. The reasons for the lower academic standard of Deakin-Warrnambool nursing graduates at this time probably had to do with the general situation of Deakin's Warrnambool campus from the early to mid-1990s. Following the closure of the teacher education course and the non-replacement or transfer of both academic and general staff, there was a general concern in the local community that the whole Warrnambool campus might close. With significant reductions in academic staff in the School of Nursing many potential students, believing that nursing at Warrnambool was likely to close, went elsewhere. Since then the situation regarding the nursing course at Warrnambool has stabilised and Deakin's nursing graduates now compete on equal terms for positions at the Hospital.

Like other employers of skilled female labour during the 1970s, the Hospital needed to develop much more flexible employment policies than previously. Traditional expectations that nurses should be single females who resided in a supervised nurses home and be prepared to work excessive hours were no longer acceptable, industrially or legally and were not in the Hospital's interest. The requirement that nurses should resign when they married had resulted in the Hospital's nursing staff consisting mainly of relatively inexperienced trainees. While nursing involved a great deal of non-nursing work, this loss of experienced nurses was partly offset by the fact that trainees provided a cheap labour force willing to work long hours. However with the ongoing increase in acute care patients the Hospital's need was for qualified, experienced nursing staff. This change in hospital policy was inevitable given the general shortage of qualified nurses, anti-discrimination legislation and general recognition of the need to increase employment opportunities for married women. In contrast to the past, married women now constitute approximately seventy per cent of the Hospital's total nursing staff.

Once responsibility for pre-service nurse education was transferred to tertiary institutions, hospitals basically lost control of the selection of trainees or student nurses which now became based on academic merit. The entry of increased numbers of males into the nursing profession in Australia is reflected in the male-female ratio of the Hospital's current nursing establishment. Whereas prior to 1972, only two English-trained male nurses were employed at the Hospital, currently around ten per cent of the Hospital's permanent nursing staff are males. The fact that more males have sought to become nurses is due to major changes in the work undertaken by qualified nursing staff. Where once nursing was closely associated with women's traditional roles as housewives and mothers, nurses are now highly skilled specialists in patient care, and paid accordingly.

Changes in the nature of work have also substantially reduced the need for state-enrolled nurses (formerly referred to as nursing aides). Much of the acute care work performed at the Hospital, in line with legal as well as clinical requirements, must be undertaken by registered nurses, preferably with specialist qualifications. By 1999, only 4.5 per cent of the Hospital's total nursing staff were state-enrolled nurses.

Indeed, in order to enhance their prospects of job security and promotion, it has now become common practice for registered nurses wishing to be employed at the Hospital to undertake postgraduate qualifications in specialised areas of nursing. Until the late 1980s, relevant experience was deemed sufficient for registered nurses involved in most acute care work. This is no longer the case and the Hospital strongly encourages nurses to complete postgraduate courses through combination of on-campus and distance education units. Warrnambool-based nurses studying in the specialist areas can also undertake eight week periods of clinical practice at Melbourne's metropolitan hospitals including St Vincents, Royal Melbourne and Box Hill. Around eighty per cent of nurses involved in specialist work at the Hospital currently hold postgraduate qualifications.

Another significant change in nursing during the nineties has been the growth of the Hospital's outreach community service, with its focus on treating patients in their homes where possible. Apart from the obvious cost savings, given the facilities of the modern home the "hospital without walls" concept is preferred by many patients and reduces the risk of the patient contracting infections in hospitals. As part of a postnatal care programme, a midwifery nurse visits mothers. Apart from the District Nursing Service, nurses with specialised skills in palliative and post-acute care are part of the Hospital's current outreach service. Though the extension of this service has required the Hospital to purchase and maintain additional cars and mobile phones, it is clearly the way of the future in terms of the Hospital responding to patients' changing needs and its own continuing financial constraints.

The development of nursing at South West Healthcare over the next ten years will presumably involve a continuation of the main changes identified in this chapter. Like primary teaching, the Hospital's nursing workforce will be relatively stable — and will consist of well qualified, experienced career nurses. Nurses are likely to be more involved in preventive health care and undertake more community and school visits as part of the Hospital's public education role. As nurses become more highly qualified and experienced, the proposed development of the nurse practitioner model will provide new career opportunities for nurses in Warrnambool and elsewhere in Victoria's south-west.

[1] *Standard*, 15 January 1986.

[2] *Standard*, 20 September 1988.

[3] *Standard*, 30 September 1986.

[4] WDBH Annual Report, 1988–89, pp.15.

[5] See WDBH Annual Reports, 1973–74 and 1997–98.

[6] In fact Dr Scott was not a specialist obstetrician as, like several local GPs, he held a diploma in obstetrics.

[7] Much of the information in this section is based on discussions with Ms Sue Morrison, director of nursing, Warrnambool Base Hospital and Ms Pat Nesbitt, senior lecturer, School of Nursing, Faculty of Health and Behavioural Sciences, Deakin University.

[8] *Standard*, 24 September 1983.

Chapter 20

MERGERS, CLOSURES AND AMALGAMATIONS: LYNDOCH, BRIERLY AND SOUTH WEST HEALTHCARE

During the 1990s the Warrnambool Base Hospital was involved in a number of major organisational changes as part of its evolution into a multi-campus institution and key provider of a broad range of health care services for south-western Victoria. Though local factors were important, amalgamations, closures and mergers were basically part of the inevitable process of modernisation and rationalisation of Australia's public hospital system. These changes reflected a rapid growth in patient demand for hospitals to provide more cost effective, specialised medical and outreach services. In the case of Victoria's public hospitals these changes were largely a response to the State Government's reforms of the public health system during the 1990s. During this period the Hospital's board of management was required to respond to the regionalisation and rationalisation of publicly funded health services in Victoria or face reductions in government funding. As part of this process the Hospital became involved in a proposed amalgamation with Lyndoch Hospital for the Aged, the takeover and subsequent closure of the Brierly Mental Hospital and the subsequent expansion of regional psychiatric services in south-west Victoria, and the establishment of South West Healthcare and the regional voluntary alliance of rural hospitals. The proposed merger with Lyndoch and the closure of Brierly generated considerable controversy in the Warrnambool community. This was not the case in the late 1990s with the merger of what had been the Warrnambool Base Hospital, and Camperdown and Lismore District Hospitals to form a new, multi-campus organisation, South West Healthcare. Nor has South West Healthcare's key role in the recent development of a voluntary alliance of fourteen public hospitals in the wider region generated much by way of public controversy or local media interest.

The 1990s probably represented the most dynamic period of change in the Hospital's one hundred and fifty year history as the board responded to major policy developments introduced by successive state governments designed to make Victoria's public hospital system more cost effective and efficient. This process usually involved the State Government commissioning then acting on the recommendations of consultants' reports into the future provision and funding of certain aspects of health services. As part of the rationalisation process several smaller country hospitals in south-west Victoria were either closed or had a much reduced role in the provision of acute health care. The closure of hospitals such as Mortlake and District Hospital was obviously significant in the Warrnambool Base Hospital's evolution as the region's major health provider. The ultimately unsuccessful attempt in 1992 to amalgamate Lyndoch Hospital for the Aged with the Base Hospital and the closure of the Brierly Mental Hospital in 1994 were both responses to the State Government's policy to modernise and rationalise Victoria's public hospital system rather than a strategy on the part of the Hospital management to take over these institutions.

Before describing these changes in greater detail it is worth noting how the Base Hospital's recent history reflects Warrnambool's development as the major regional centre for south-west Victoria. Until the 1960s Warrnambool was the largest of a number of cities in the region, which included Hamilton and Portland with populations of around 10,000, as well as smaller towns such as Port Fairy, Mortlake, Terang and Camperdown with populations of less than 4,000. However with the development of cheaper, more reliable motor transport and the growth of public demand for more sophisticated services, including medical services, Warrnambool-Port Fairy has become the major and only growth centre for the region while the populations of other towns have declined. Within the south-west there is some feeling of resentment towards Warrnambool as a so-called "sponge centre" which is allegedly draining people and resources from the rest of the region. Such attitudes, though difficult to quantify, need to be taken into account in understanding the Hospital's evolution since 1972 from what was essentially a town and local district community hospital to an administratively complex, multi-campus regional provider of health services.

To explain why the former State Labor Government's proposal to amalgamate Lyndoch with the Base Hospital generated such a hostile response within the local community we need to understand something of Lyndoch's history. It was established as an *old folks home* in 1952 following the purchase of land near the Hopkins River by local builder, Ern Harris. The management and subsequent development of Lyndoch were very much community based. The dominant figure in Lyndoch's impressive growth was the local identity, Stan Berlyn, who joined the committee of management on 12 May 1952. According to Peter Yule, the author of a recent history of Lyndoch, Berlyn, who became Vice President and Treasurer in 1960, "for the next twenty-five years ran Lyndoch like an absolute monarch"[1]. With Ern Harris, Stan Berlyn presided over Lyndoch's expansion, which included a major building programme, until the two had a falling out when Harris's firm was not awarded a contract to build the new Lyndoch Day Hospital in 1970. For reasons which are not altogether clear, but possibly related to Berlyn's dominant style of leadership, the relationship between the Base Hospital and Lyndoch was neither cooperative nor cordial. This situation apparently improved in 1984 when Dr Noel Bayley was appointed as a geriatrician at Lyndoch. The appointment of local GP, Dr Mike Page, who succeeded Stan Berlyn as President of the Lyndoch Board in October 1987, is seen by Peter Yule as the beginning of a new era. However in 1989 an external report presented to the Lyndoch Board of Management on 14 August by the Canadian expert Professor Ronald Cope noted that "collaboration between Lyndoch and the Warrnambool Base Hospital could be increased and improved"[2].

In 1991 the then Labor State Government initiated a push to amalgamate Victoria's aged care and acute care hospitals. Following a report by the health care consultant Ross Naylor, the then Minister for Health, Maureen Lister, announced the Government's intention to amalgamate Lyndoch and the Base Hospital. This was rightly perceived by some local opponents of the move as part of the Government's programme to cut costs to help resolve a budget crisis. The considerable opposition within the Warrnambool community was led by Councillor David Atkinson and the National Party Member for Warrnambool, John McGrath. However while Naylor's report stated that the merger would save an estimated $317,000 per year, it also emphasised the benefits to patients which would include increased "provision of a broad range of aged care services in Warrnambool"[3].

Responding to Naylor's report which recommended the amalgamation officially start on 1 July 1991 John McGrath argued that "Lyndoch [was] a very efficient institution receiving outstanding support from the Warrnambool community . . . this could be in jeopardy if the merger goes ahead"[4].

Led by McGrath and the chairman of the Lyndoch Combined Anti-Amalgamation Lobby, Neil McDonald, the opponents of amalgamation held a protest meeting on 15 January in Warrnambool and subsequently demonstrated on the steps of Parliament House in Melbourne on April 28 in 1992. This renewed activity early in 1992 was a response to the leaking of a draft report to the Minister for Health, Maureen Lister, which recommended that the amalgamation should proceed. According to John McGrath in an article published in the *Standard* on 4 April 1992, "the draft report would spark World War III in Warrnambool". Apart from arguments that Lyndoch was already a highly efficient operation and would lose community support if the amalgamation proceeded, Lyndoch officials raised the prospect of net job losses if the merger went ahead. According to the CEO, Rex Spencer, "staff cuts were expected if the merger proceeded with reductions in several highly paid positions a certainty"[5]. At this stage Mr Spencer's own employment prospects were not of concern as he was due to retire the next month. The State Government made it clear that no replacement CEO would be appointed until the amalgamation issue was finalised.

In publicly supporting the amalgamation proposal, the Hospital's board of management found itself allied with a now unpopular State Government, firmly opposed by Lyndoch management and supporters' groups, the local council and a popular local member of Parliament. Like the State Government, the Hospital's reasons for supporting Ross Naylor's recommendations were based on the view the amalgamation would resolve and improve patient care and bring cost savings. According to the Hospital's CEO Peter McGregor, "savings achieved could be reallocated to direct patient care services for the benefit of the Warrnambool community"[6]. The amalgamation proposal produced a generally hostile response which included a double page of letters to the *Standard* on 8 July 1992, all of which opposed the merger. One of these letters was from Dr Ian Pettigrew; writing as chairman of the south-west division of the AMA he indicated that there was little support for the merger from local doctors. According to Dr Pettigrew "while accepting that there may be benefits to the Base Hospital, there has, to date, been little evidence to suggest that Lyndoch and its clientele would benefit"[7]. Dr John Christie, Director of Medical Services at the Hospital, responded to Dr Pettigrew's comments in a detailed letter to the *Standard* published on 14 July 1992 where he restated the Board's reason for supporting the merger and expressed hope that "this debate will not degenerate into an irrational, emotive diatribe of allegations or half truths". In their letter to the *Standard*, Doctors Noel Bayley and Michael Page took issue with a number of points raised in Dr Christie's letter which they claimed included "significantly incomplete quoting" from key reports, concluding that "if the proposal has to be assessed on its merits . . . it must now be judged as failed".

In the face of community and political opposition, the Minister Maureen Lister's decision not to proceed was hardly surprising. The Minister's letter guaranteeing that the amalgamation would not proceed regardless of the result of the forthcoming election was presented to Lyndoch's Acting CEO Frank O'Brien by the ALP candidate for Warrnambool John Thomson. Clearly the ALP was hoping that this gesture would improve the Labor candidate's prospects in the forthcoming state election.

BRIERLY

The dust had barely settled on the Lyndoch amalgamation issue when the threatened closure of Brierly Mental Hospital again involved the Hospital management in a major public controversy. Established in 1957, Brierly occupied approximately sixty-eight acres to the north-east of Warrnambool and was a traditional country town mental asylum. The Base Hospital had taken over the administration of Brierly, unlike Lyndoch, in 1991. In retrospect Brierly's closure and the subsequent establishment of a regional community-based psychiatric services organisation were inevitable both for financial and medical reasons. There had been major changes in the delivery of psychiatric services and a traditional mental hospital like Brierly was viewed by government and the medical profession as inefficient and archaic. Following its election in October 1992, the Kennett Coalition

State Government was determined to reduce public expenditure on health services significantly. Its budget-oriented health policies involved the replacement of expensive public mental hospitals with cheaper, community-based mental health programmes. This reform was very much in keeping with the national health policy which had been endorsed by the state ministers for health in April 1992. Like the Lyndoch amalgamation proposal, the controversy which subsequently arose over the proposed closure of Brierly reflected deep-seated suspicion within the local community and among Brierly staff that this was basically a cost cutting initiative with little regard for the interest of patients, Brierly's employees or the local community.

The integration of the Warrnambool Base Hospital and the new regional Glenelg Psychiatric Services on 1 April 1992 clearly committed the Hospital management to the eventual closure of Brierly. On 2 April 1991 an item in the *Standard* announced that Brierly would close in mid-1996 and that this would involve the loss of sixty-seven jobs.[8] An announcement by the minister for health that Victoria's public hospitals would have to absorb an 11.9 per cent budget cut over two years ensured that this deadline would be implemented. The board's reasons for wishing to close Brierly in the face of considerable local opposition were obvious enough. As one of the Hospital's current senior managers explained, Brierly Hospital was perceived as something of a sheltered workshop — poorly managed and overstaffed — which provided a discredited form of care for mental patients. A community-based regional system of psychiatric services was seen as more equitable as it would provide improved services to south-west Victoria's population of over 100,000 people.

The two major sources of public opposition to the planned closure of Brierly were a community-based group — the Warrnambool Association for the Support of Psychiatric Services — and the Health and Community Services Union. The Association, which supported the change to community-based care for the mentally ill, produced a study which was critical of the Hospital's business plan for the future provision of psychiatric services for the region. This study was sceptical of certain aspects of the Hospital's claims that the level of patient care would be improved while implementing significant budget cuts. Co-author of the study, Brenda Harrison, a lecturer in nursing at Deakin University, claimed that the Hospital's business plan was driven by "economic rationalist points of view rather than motivated by genuine concern for sufferers' and carers' needs"[9]. According to Kaye Williams, the state secretary of the Health and Community Services Union, the proposed changes reflected the Kennett Government's hard line economic policies rather than a desire to improve the quality of patient care. In Ms Williams' view "the guts were being ripped out of the psychiatric services in the south-west"[10].

The decision to close Brierly and implement regional, community-based psychiatric services was strongly defended by Dr Dennis Napthine as parliamentary secretary to the minister for health and MLA for Portland, and Andrew Rowe on behalf of the Hospital's board. According to Dr Napthine the changes "were clearly not cost driven" and " the whole move to community based care and mainstreaming [moving psychiatric patients into general hospitals] . . . is best for people with psychiatric illnesses". In Dr Napthine's view "we shouldn't be providing funding to inefficient hospitals to provide jobs for people when there are people on the waiting list for treatment"[11].

Another critic of the planned closure of Brierly was Joan Grace, the Head Supervisor of the Francis Foundation, a non-profit organisation which provided accommodation for local people with psychiatric illnesses. According to Mrs Grace, most "clients, who had relocated to Brierly over the past years find this is like their lifeline being cut"[12]. Responding to the claims that the closure of Brierly was being driven by economic rationalism and represented a significant downgrading of mental health services in the region, the Hospital's CEO Andrew Rowe wrote a carefully-worded letter to the *Standard* published on 3 April 1993. As well as outlining specific benefits including the "increased number of professional staff to work in the community" Mr Rowe's letter provided details of "a specifically designed acute psychiatric services unit to be constructed on the Hospital's Ryot St complex". The public controversy over Brierly died down quickly, though the future use of the Brierly site remains unresolved.

SOUTH WEST HEALTHCARE

In contrast to the attempted amalgamation with Lyndoch and the closure of Brierly, the June 1999 merger between the Warrnambool Base Hospital and Corangamite Health Services to form South West Healthcare was well received by both communities involved. From the start, it was obvious that the proposed amalgamation was in the interest of both organisations with the Warrnambool Hospital's management determined to ensure that the process did not result in organised opposition from the smaller communities of Camperdown, Lismore and Derrinallum. Discussions and the official agreements that preceded the official merger address the obvious concern of these communities that their hospitals were being taken over by the Base Hospital and that this would result in a reduction of patient services. In a discussion in October 1998 the boards of both organisations agreed that the following "significant benefits" could be achieved through a full amalgamation:

- improved health planning;
- sharing of IT resources;
- additional ability to recruit and retain key professional staff by offering greater career paths and prospects;
- integration so that all required services could be accessed from one point of entry regardless of location;
- computer networking of services;

- enhanced medical recruitment, retention and training relevant to general practitioners and specialists;
- greater integration and coordination of care through case management;
- enhanced access to a vast array of expertise and services by both organisations;
- ongoing development of primary care, maternity services, discharge planning, Hospital in the Home and post acute care, etc.;
- consistency with government and DHS policy and the support of both local parliamentarians and the minister for health.

They also considered the amalgamation:

- capable of being achieved without acrimony;
- likely to be supported by the communities involved; and
- able to provide a blue print for future developments in south-west Victoria and provides a model for similar initiatives in other rural regions.[13]

Both organisations had previous experience of mergers, with the Corangamite Regional Hospital Services having been established on 1 January 1995 from an amalgamation of the Camperdown and District and Lismore District Hospitals, and the Lismore and Derrinallum Nursing Home Society. As well as stating that the amalgamation would provide "a significant opportunity for both organisations and the communities they serve" the crucial Heads of Agreement document sought to reassure both patients and doctors in the smaller centres that their interests would be protected. As well as guaranteeing that the "retention [and] enhancement of core patient care services delivered at each site shall be a priority for the new agency" the document stated that the "new organisation will strive to maintain, encourage and enhance the role of general practitioners"[14]. This

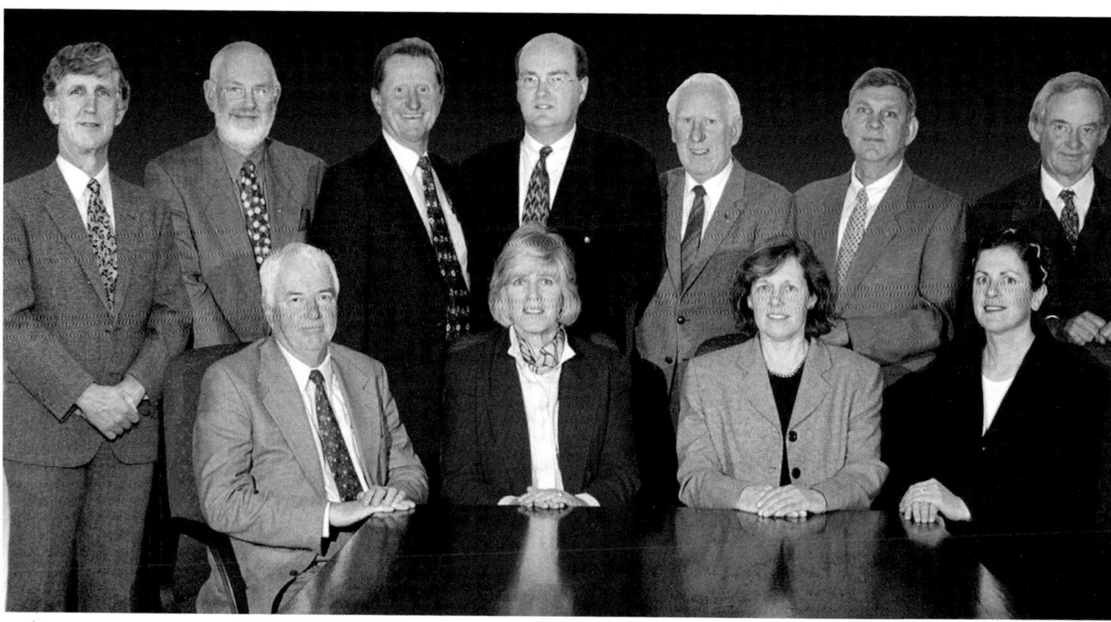

South West Healthcare board of management. Standing: Dr J. Menzies, Mr J.E. Wilson, Snr Sgt I. Armstrong, Mr D.R. Jellie, Mr J. Clark, Mr P. Roysland, Dr K.D. Nunn. Seated: Mr S. Carroll, Barbara Piesse, Mrs V. Lang, Mrs J. McKenzie, 1999–2000.

proposed agreement also stipulated that "subject to approval from the minister" in the new agency's board of management, eight of the new representatives would be from Warrnambool and four from Corangamite, with "each organisation responsible for nominating the respective members in accordance with the above allocations". The name of the new organisation, South West Healthcare, was chosen from a list of four options which included Southern Coast Health and Warrnambool/Corangamite Health. Once the August 1998 heads of agreement had been approved by both boards of management it was submitted for formal approval to the regional director, Barwon South Western Region, to take effect from 1 July 1999.

At the time of the merger, Warrnambool Base Hospital and Corangamite Regional Hospital Services were potentially complementary organisations. For a start, Warrnambool with a total of 180 available beds (156 acute care, twenty-five psychiatric services) was approximately two and a half times the size of Corangamite Regional Hospital Services with its 69.5 beds, only thirty-one of which were acute care with twenty-eight nursing home and eight hostel beds. In accordance with State Government policy, following the closure of Corio House, Warrnambool Base Hospital had transferred its aged care beds to the private sector, with the Moran Health Care Group the successful tenderer. With the extensive community outreach programme, Warrnambool's total staffing level in 1997/98 of 495.11 equivalent positions was almost seven times that of the Corangamite Regional Hospital Services (69.5). Following the official announcement of the merger on 1 July 1999 there has been no indication, at least in the local press, that the new arrangements under South West Healthcare have been other than successful.

[1] Peter Yule, "History of Lyndoch," unpublished manuscript.
[2] *Standard*, 26 June 1992.
[3] Ibid.
[4] *Standard*, 3 June 1991.
[5] *Standard*, 4 April 1992.
[6] *Standard*, 4 April 1992.
[7] *Standard*, 8 July 1992.
[8] *Standard*, 2 April 1991.
[9] *Standard*, 5 June 1993.
[10] Ibid.
[11] Ibid.
[12] Ibid.
[13] Discussion with DHS, 23 October 1998.
[14] Heads of Agreement, Warrnambool and District Base Hospital and the Corangamite Regional Hospital Service, dated 26 August 1998.

Chapter 21

THE SOUTH WEST ALLIANCE OF RURAL HOSPITALS: CONCLUSION

Following shortly after the Warrnambool Hospital's merger with Corangamite Regional Health Service to form the multi-campus South West Healthcare in October 1997, Warrnambool was the largest of twelve public hospitals to formally commit staff to membership of the newly established South West Alliance of Rural Hospitals (SWARH). In terms of the Hospital's history this State Coalition Government initiative was part of the process whereby once autonomous public hospitals become part of increasingly integrated regional health care services. In 1997 the Department of Health Services, after consultation by KPMG, introduced its Information, Information Technology and Telecommunications Strategy (I2T2) as a means of developing a more cost efficient and effective system of publicly funded health care in Victoria. The State Government announced an annual 1.5 per cent reduction in Victoria's acute care public hospitals' budget based on expected productivity savings arising from investment in I2T2. KPMG's report suggested investment required to gain these savings was $400 million over four years. The actual investment made by the Department was only 25 per cent or $100 million over a four year period (1997–2001). To have access to this money, regional hospitals such as Warrnambool Base were required to become part of larger voluntary alliances of rural hospitals. Each grouping was to have a technical leader with a steering group consisting of the CEOs of member hospitals. The metropolitan public hospitals were required by the State Government to form themselves into networks with a single CEO and effectively a single multi-site organisation.

It was the government's intention to utilise improved telecommunications technology to substantially change the culture and practices of Victoria's public hospitals as "autonomous health services with little peer interaction or . . . substantive resource sharing between organisations"[1]. While participation of public hospitals in the I2T2 strategy was "voluntary" there were strong financial incentives for hospitals such as Warrnambool to join these voluntary alliances. The State Government divided Victoria into fourteen new health regions, the south-west being one of five rural regions. As well as anticipated cost savings through investment in IT infrastructure, the Government's agenda was to increase access to patient information between health organisations (mainly hospitals) across regions and across the state. Central to the rationale of this strategy was that it would enable a patient to be able to present at any organisation (hospital) and have his or her medical history, tests and associated diagnosis available to the attending clinician.

In October 1997 Warrnambool (as part of South West Healthcare) was one of twelve organisations to become part of a voluntary grouping of thirteen health services which also included the Casterton Memorial Hospital, Colac Community Health Services (Colac and Birregurra), Coleraine and District Hospital, Western District Health Services (Hamilton and Penshurst), Heywood and District Hospital, Otway Health and Community Services (Apollo Bay), Moyne Health Services (Port Fairy), Portland and District Hospital, Terang and Mortlake Health Services, Corangamite Health Services (Camperdown and Lismore) and Timboon District Hospital. Each service was to retain its own board with the CEOs forming a regional steering committee. Wary of arousing local opposition the Government made membership of alliances on the part of public hospitals quite voluntary. As a result the boundaries of the South West Alliance of Rural Hospitals were based on decisions made by particular hospital administrations rather than being aligned with existing local government or other administrative boundaries. For example while Apollo Bay Hospital (Otway Health and Community Services) decided to join the South West Alliance, the Boards of the Lorne and Winchelsea Hospital opted to be part of Barwon Region.

In June 1998 Garry Druitt, formerly IT strategic planning and client services manager Deakin University, was appointed as SWARH's chief information officer to oversee the implementation of the I2T2 strategy.

In January 1999 SWARH's steering committee signed a joint venture agreement which committed each of the organisations to the I2T2 strategy and adopted SWARH as a business name.

The steering committee engaged the consultants KPMG to develop an "Information, Information Technology and Telecommunications Strategic Plan for the South West Alliance", which was completed in September 1998. In 1996 the State Government had engaged KPMG to determine the extent to which proper utilisation of advanced information technology could improve productivity in Victoria's public hospitals. After spelling out how the I2T2 could "serve as a catalyst to enable SWARH's members to implement best practice by . . . overcoming long standing issues of timelines, distance and access" KPMG's report provided an economic rationale for the SWARH's required investment of about $20 million in IT over a five year period. [2] The key points raised in this report provide a clear indication of just how dramatically the basis of funding the future development of public hospitals, such as Warrnambool's, had changed since the 1970s.

In their report, the consultants pointed out that Victoria's public hospitals were limited in their ability to invest, as new investment is not linked to improving services which increase patient revenues. This is because under

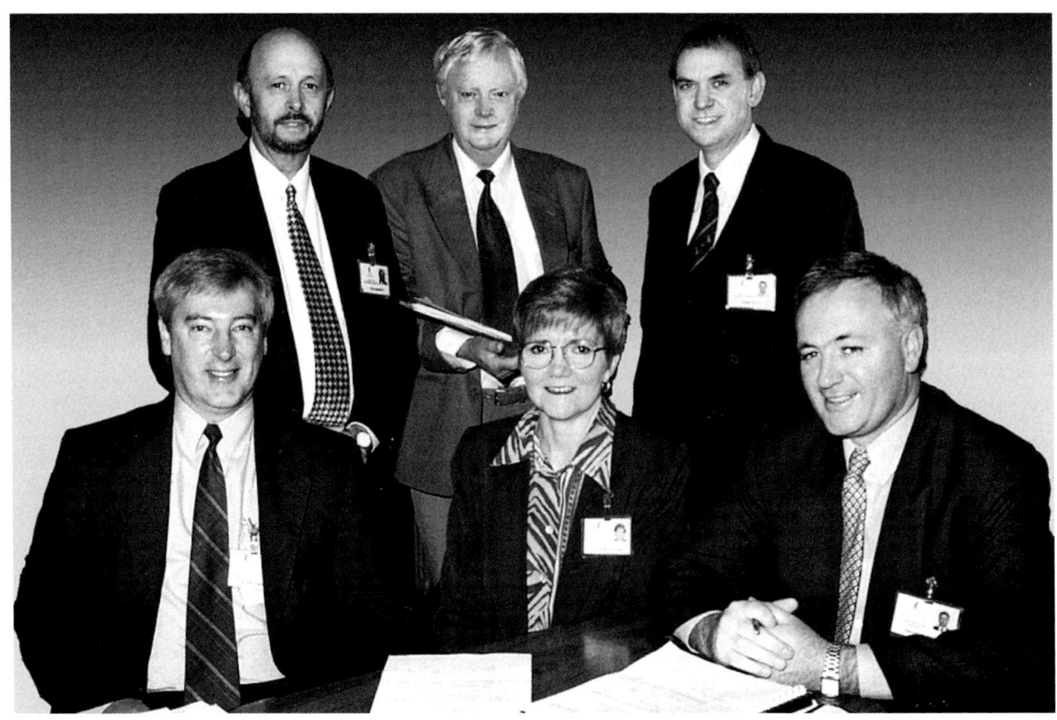

The Hospital's executive staff, 2000. From left: director of psychiatric services Mr Ken Burnett, and director of finance Mr Ian Barton. Seated from the left: director of medical services Dr Peter O'Brien, director of nursing Mrs Sue Morrison, and chief executive officer Mr Andrew Rowe, Corangamite Regional Hospital Services chief executive officer Mr Chris Scott (standing right).

the casemix funding formula the Government determines the total number of treatments and the financial value of treatments, which effectively limits the revenue of the hospitals. For a public hospital, "in the face of such fixed revenues . . . reducing cost of service delivery is the only way of creating a surplus for investment". According to the consultants, based on recent American studies, I2T2 is one of the few areas of investment with the potential to reduce significantly hospitals' costs of service delivery. The KPMG report addresses the issue of how Warrnambool- South West Healthcare together with other SWARH members could generate $11 million in cost savings of the $20 million required to warrant the required investment in I2T2. The most obvious area of direct cost savings was in reducing certain costs such as telephone calls and video conferencing. More significant were *potential* savings as a result of more efficient business practices within the Alliance.

Based on their 1996 report for the Department of Health Services, KPMG reported that the implementation of the I2T2 Strategy over a five year period should reduce the average cost of each inpatient treated by 34.1 per cent while increasing the revenue of each inpatient treated by 28.1 per cent. The consultants made the point that while the implementation of the I2T2 Strategy did not directly guarantee improved revenue or reduced cost for public hospitals such as Warrnambool it had the potential to do both. The consultants refer to the "good road" analysis. For like the I2T2 Strategy the construction of a "good road" has the potential to reduce costs and improve business for road users because it provides for the use of larger and faster vehicles.

The Hospital's Board of Management was obviously convinced by these arguments to become a fully participating and hence contributing member of the Voluntary Alliance. With the other hospital managements, the board saw its financial contribution to the I2T2 strategy as a sound financial investment on the part of the Hospital.

According to Gary Druitt, the major difficulty in achieving the I2T2 objectives will be political rather than financial or technical. For the strategy to be effectively implemented, the twelve CEOs and autonomous boards of the member organisations will need to reach general agreement regarding priorities. The fact that the largest institution involved, South West Healthcare, is more than twenty times the size of the smallest obviously created certain tensions in the decision making process.

THE FUTURE

The fundamental organisational changes that have resulted in the once largely autonomous Warrnambool and District Base Hospital becoming part of an increasingly integrated regional health care network are more real than apparent. For most Warrnambool residents, in terms of the physical appearance and perceived function of the Hospital, little has changed. Unlike the attempted amalgamation with Lyndoch or the closure of Brierly, the negotiation process which led to the South West Healthcare merger, and the formation of SWARH, generated little public controversy or even interest in the local press. Yet the Hospital has changed fundamentally since 1972 as it evolved towards becoming the largest campus in an increasingly integrated, corporatised, state government-directed regional health service.

Warrnambool, like other former regional base hospitals, has changed and will continue to change in the type of services offered and how these are to be provided. As advanced societies move towards the creation of the virtual hospital, improved communications technology and highly trained staff rather than buildings will be the critical infrastructure required. Consistent trends evident during the past three decades, with the Hospital treating increased numbers of acute care inpatients for shorter periods, will continue. Public hospitals such as Warrnambool's will be expected to take increased responsibility for preventive health care and will be funded accordingly. While regional hospitals will continue to be where local people go to receive specialised medical treatment, these institutions will increasingly become facilitators of diverse health care services. With both the State and Federal Governments regarding health care as just another service, publicly-funded providers like Warrnambool Hospital will be required to compete with private providers for government funding. Yet, as has been the case with Warrnambool Hospital, with its corporate management structure and business practices, and privatisation of certain departments, the once clear cut division between public and private hospitals will be increasingly blurred.

Older members of the Warrnambool community, including certain local doctors and other individuals with a long association with the Hospital, may experience a sense of regret at what has been lost as a result of the changes outlined above. What was Warrnambool Base Hospital is no longer the community-based institution it once was. Yet given the population of south-west Victoria's ever growing demand for increased, better quality, yet affordable and locally accessible health services, these changes were both inevitable and desirable. It is to be hoped that this history will assist the regional community to understand better how and why changes in the Hospital's development over the past century and a half have taken place.

[1] Notes provided by the SWARH chief information officer, Gary Druitt, presentation 1999.
[2] KPMG, South West Alliance of Rural Hospitals: Information, Information Technology and Telecommunications Strategic Plan, September 1998, executive summary — update 2000, p.5.

APPENDIX Details of Interviews

Individuals are listed in the order in which interviews were conducted. Individuals interviewed were selected from a list provided by the Hospital executive.

Dr Kevin Longton	general practitioner
Mr Bill Wines	former patient and volunteer
Mrs Thelma Surridge	former trainee and nurse
Mr Richard Ziegler	occupational therapist 1970–90
Mrs J.P Moore	past president, Warrnambool Hospital Auxiliary
Mrs Agnes Kent	former trainee and nurse
Mrs Rita Brauer	former trainee and nurse and wife of Dr A. Brauer
Mr Brian Dillon	director, Hospital pharmacy, 1987–97
Mrs Elsie Smith	former patient
Mr Jim Henry	whose parents provided milk for the Hospital
Mrs Joan Houlahan	former trainee and currently a nurse at the Hospital
Miss June Stewart	former matron
Ms Karen Lindford	Nestles Sports and Social Club
Mrs Judy Ross	Woolsthorpe Auxiliary
Ms Sue Morrison	director of nursing
Dr Harry Savery	general practitioner
Mrs Helen Chislett	Naringal Auxiliary
Mr Rex Johnson	former engineer
Mr John Reid	pathologist 1964–84
Mr Gary Weeks	former director of pharmacy
Mrs Irene Bruce	
Ms Helen Wilson	coordinator, Centre Against Sexual Assault
Ms Patricia Nesbitt	School of Nursing, Deakin University
Mr John Norton	former board member
Mr Eric Fairbanks	general practitioner, director of Palliative Care Unit
Mr Ken Burnett	director, psychiatric services
Mrs June Foster	former pharmacy assistant
Mr Peter OBrien	director of medical services
Dr James Rossiter	paediatrician 1964–68
Mr Stephen Fischer	general surgeon
Mr Frank Lodge	past president and Hospital board member
Dr Roger Brough	drug and alcohol physician
Ms Barbara Piesse	president of the Hospital board
Ms Margaret Woodford	former nurse trainee
Dr Chris Beaton	obstetrician/gynaecologist
Dr Les Hemingway	general practitioner
Mr Gary Druitt	chief information officer, South West Alliance of Rural Hospitals
Dr David Shimmins	general practitioner
Mr Andrew Rowe	Chief executive officer, South West Healthcare

Index